AIDS IN AFRICA

An African
and
Prophetic Perspective

Foreword by Ambassador Mary Kanya

By

Rev. Dr. Mankekolo Mahlangu-Ngcobo, MPH

Gateway Press, Inc.
Baltimore, Maryland
2001

Cover art drawn by Khotso Kale, 16 year old South African.

Copyright © 2001 by Rev. Dr. Mankekolo Mahlangu-Ngcobo, MPH
All rights reserved.

Permission to reproduce in any form must be secured in writing from the author.

Please direct all correspondence and book orders to:
Rev. Dr. Mankekolo Mahlangu-Ngcobo
3315 Mondawmin Ave.
Baltimore, MD 21215
email: Mankekolo@aol.com
Bookstore/Wholesale inquiries, please call or FAX (410) 233-4649

ISBN 0-9652001-5-9

Published for the author by
Gateway Press, Inc.
1001 N. Calvert St.
Baltimore, MD 21202

Printed in the United States of America

DEDICATION

This book is dedicated, first, to persons who came into my life professionally and through the ministry, who died of AIDS, and to all others who have died of AIDS.

This book is also dedicated to those who are HIV positive, and to people who are living with AIDS. To individuals, families, NGOs, governments, faith communities, and international organizations who are engaged in the "war" to prevent HIV infection and care for persons—babies and the young and old— living with AIDS.

Lastly, this book is dedicated to those who are praying for and researching for a cure for AIDS.

TABLE OF CONTENTS

Foreword vii
Acknowledgements ix
Preface x

1. Africa—Sweet Home 1
2. The ABC of Viruses, HIV and AIDS 5
3. Human Immune Deficiency Virus Is Preventable 15
4. The Role of the African Family 21
5. The Role of the African Non-Governmental Organization 28
6. The Role of the African Government 34
7. The Role of the African Faith Communities 39
8. The Role of the International Communities 48
9. A Prophetic Serman on Mt. Kilimanjaro 52
10. A Prayer for Africa 57

Appendix A: Excerpt from HIV/AIDS Population Impact Chart 61
Notes 64
About the Author 66

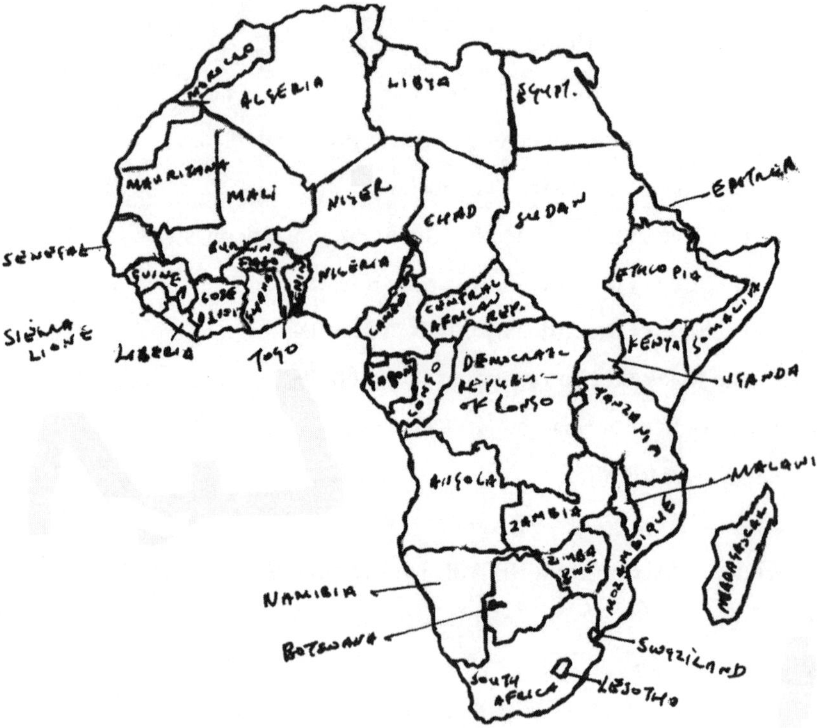
ALGERIA
LIBYA
EGYPT.
ERITREA
MAURITANIA
MALI
NIGER
CHAD
SUDAN
SENEGAL
NIGERIA
ETHIOPIA
CENTRAL AFRICAN REP.
SOMALIA
KENYA
UGANDA
SIERRA LEONE
LIBERIA
TOGO
CONGO
TANZANIA
ANGOLA
MALAWI
ZAMBIA
MOZAMBIQUE
MADAGASCAR
NAMIBIA
BOTSWANA
SWAZILAND
SOUTH AFRICA
LESOTHO

FOREWORD

I am honored to be asked to write the foreword of a thoughtful, challenging and inspiring book on AIDS in Africa from the African and prophetic perspective.

There cannot be any doubt that the HIV/AIDS epidemic has presented the world with one of the most devastating threats to humankind in recent memory and Africa continues to be the most affected. It is my belief that no family in Africa, Sub-Saharan Africa in particular, has been left untouched by HIV/AIDS.

Millions of children have been orphaned by this epidemic. The psycho-social impact of the disease on the orphaned children is beginning to unfold in Sub-Saharan Africa. As the children drop out of school, either to care for their dying parents, or to fend for themselves, the number of street children increases. This is most likely to result in an upsurge of criminal activity and civil unrest.

Rev. Dr. Mahlangu-Ngcobo reminds us of the cultural strength of the African extended family. She suggests that the family should be empowered educationally, morally and financially to care for family members living with AIDS.

Gains that had been achieved over decades in controlling infectious childhood diseases by immunization have been lost in few years due to the pandemic. In fact, mortality rates are already on the increase.

Indeed, the reduction in life expectancy in most affected areas has been very drastic. In some Southern African countries, the average life expectancy has been reduced by more than 20 years because of HIV/AIDS.

As the disease continues to hit the most economically productive group of society, the economies of African countries are beginning to suffer irreparable damage.

The negative impact of the HIV/AIDS epidemic on economic productivity, regional stability and security in Sub-Saharan Africa is likely to affect the Western economies in the years to come.

At the beginning of this new millennium it is indeed worrisome that the less developed world continues to bear the brunt of the epidemic.

As our African continent struggles to find solution to this pandemic, Rev. Dr. Mahlangu-Ngcobo prophetically brings the SPIRIT OF HOPE. She offers African culturally sensitive, collaborative and comprehensive ideas to individuals, families, non-governmental organizations, governments, faith communities, business communities and international agencies to stop the incidence of HIV infection and reduce the prevalence of AIDS.

Bear in mind this disease respects no borders. We should all strive together and engage all resources at our disposal to arrest the spread of the pandemic. Let us remember that the world is now a global village, and whatever befalls one community should galvanize us all to action. Failure to contain this epidemic in Africa will inevitably affect the whole of humanity.

Fortunately, Rev. Dr. Mankekolo Mahlangu-Ngcobo in this wonderful book gives us the inspiration and the wisdom, which leads us to the path of HOPE, HELP and HEALING.

Her Excellency Mary Kanya
The Kingdom of Swaziland, Ambassador to the U.S.

ACKNOWLEDGMENTS

I am extremely grateful for the support of my sister-friend, Dr. Michele Rigaud, founder and CEO of Partners in Health and Director of the HIV Prevention program of the Health Education and Resources Organization (HERO) for critically reading the manuscript and providing resources for typing it.

My greatest gratitude is to Her Excellency Mary Kanya, the Swaziland Ambassador to the United States of America for writing the Foreword for this book.

I would like to thank sincerely the following individuals: Professor R. Omotayo Olaniyan, Economic Advisor of the Organization of African Unity (OAU), Permanent Observer Mission to the United Nations, Dr. and Mrs. Buti, Mmasello Kale, Legal Advisor of the United Nations High Commission for Refugees, Brother and Sister in Christ, Mr. and Dr. Luc, Anick Chebou, and Dr. Jules Kouatchou, for their support in writing this book.

I would also like to thank Ann Hughes for editing and publishing this book.

Thank you Ms. Lise Mohle for typing the first draft. Thank you, Kalafong A.M.E. Mission Church for praying for me. Thank you to my son, Lovey Rantjawe, and his family, and to my daughter Ntokozo, for encouraging me always.

PREFACE

"AIDS in Africa." There are headlines on television screens, newspaper pages, internet sites, and on radio broadcasts. As I read news about AIDS in Africa, I wanted to understand if what I read was true. I called some people at my home in South Africa. I asked many Africans from other African countries and they told me that it was true that young people were dying of AIDS. These people now continue to ask me, as someone who was born in Africa and now lives in the United States, "What can I do?"

I read many reactions: the criticisms of President Thabo Mbeki's statement that poverty is the root cause, at the opening of the World Conference on AIDS in Durban, 2000; Nkosi Johnson, a little boy suffering from AIDS, who stood and spoke up so that people would understand that people with AIDS are human beings; the challenges the South African government is facing to provide HIV antiretroviral drugs to pregnant women; the legal battle between the pharmaceutical companies, South Africa and AIDS activists on access to antiretroviral drugs; the fear, anger, anxiety and hopelessness of the masses, who do not understand the cause of the disease; the denial and politicization of the epidemic by some African leaders; the acceptance of HIV and AIDS as adevastating disease with many repercussions including destruction of the family by some governments; the efforts of some governments and non-governmental organizations in prevention and clinical care; the competition in funding between AIDS and for other preventable and curable diseases such as malaria, TB, and cholera; the international support needed to assist African countries with funds for development; and the difficult position of the church to be prophetic or compassionate or both. Several papers suggested that Africa would be devastated by the impact of AIDS by 2020. The United Nations General Secretary Kofi Annan had a conference with Heads of State of the Organization of African Unity in Abuja in April, 2001, in Nigeria. Another Special Session of the General Assembly of the United Nations was held in June at the United Nations Headquarters in New York to discuss public policies and find solutions and resources for AIDS in Africa.

The question I had to ask myself was: "What can I do as an African born, public health professional, author, activist, mother and pastor?" I decided to write this book, as a contribution to how we can scheme against an HIV virus that is harmless outside the human body but destructive inside the human body.

This book is not about whether HIV causes AIDS, or where HIV or AIDS originated from or if there is a conspiracy. These questions are certainly relevant and need to be studied and explored. However, this book is about the enemy number one, human immunodeficiency virus (HIV), what it is and how we can, as individuals, families, communities, governments, religious organizations, businesses, health care providers, non-governmental organizations in Africa, international governments, non-governmental organizations and churches abroad, can fight HIV and AIDS. How can we work together and not compete with each other or blame each other to prevent the HIV infection and AIDS and reduce the incidence rate (the number of new cases)?

The first chapter will explore the context of Africa. When we say AIDS in Africa, what and who is Africa? Chapter 2 will discuss HIV, the agent, what are the modes of transmission, and screening and ethical issues, AIDS, the disease, the signs and symptoms and the emotional impact on persons with AIDS. Chapter 3 will discuss the personal responsibility, especially as it pertains to sexual behavior. Chapter 4 will discuss the family response to AIDS and relatives who are infected with HIV and have AIDS. Chapter 5 will discuss the role of non-government organizations in the prevention of HIV. Chapter 6 will discuss the challenges of the African governments' public policies in linking prevention and care of those affected and infected with HIV. Chapter 7 will explore the prophetic and compassionate role of religious organizations. Chapter 8 will discuss the empowering role of the international bodies, governmental and non-governmental, and missions from abroad. In Chapter 10, I will share the Sermon on Mt. Kilimanjaro. I will close the book with the prayer for all of us in Chapter 11

There are issues that the reader may agree or disagree with. It is all right if we disagree, but we must not bicker and lose focus on the enemy—HIV and AIDS. My intention is to bring help, healing, and hope during this epidemic, from the African and prophetic perspective.

While research is going on to find vaccines or drugs to prevent and cure AIDS, we can depend on the power within us to keep HIV outside the human body. HIV is not curable now, but it is PREVENTABLE if we have the knowledge to change attitudes and behaviors. Maatla ke a rona (Sesotho, Setswana, Sepedi). Amandla ngawethu (isiZulu, IsiXhosa). Tukuna nguvu (Swahili). Ayinwere ike' (Ibo). We have the power. We shall conquer HIV and AIDS the same way we did with Colonialism and Apartheid.

CHAPTER 1

Africa – Sweet Home

Africa is not a state or province, Africa is not a country. Africa is a continent with 53 countries. In 1999, the population was 778.4 million according to the World Bank data. The land area is 29, 367 (thousands of square km.). According to the latest data of the World Bank, some 300 million Africans live on barely 65 cents a day. The Average Growth National Product (GNP) per capita for the region is US$492, but in 24 countries GNP per capita is under US$350. The lowest GNP per capita is found in African countries in conflict, for example Ethiopia (US$100), The Democratic Republic of Congo (US$110), Burundi (US$120) and Sierra Leone (US$130). There is growing urbanization. It is expected that the urban population will outnumber the people living in the rural areas by 2025. In Nigeria, Kenya and Tanzania, there are now twice as many people, living in urban centers today than 20 years ago. The percentage has tripled in Mozambique. Child mortality is a problem in Africa. Infant mortality is close to 100 per 1000 births. On average, 151 of every 1000 die before the age of 5. In many countries the infant mortality rate exceeds 200 per 1000. Life expectancy is declining since the HIV/AIDS epidemic. There is more progress in literacy than in health. The enrollment of girls in high school has doubled even though it is lagging behind the boys.

Africa is divided into five regions: Southern Africa, Eastern Africa, Middle Africa, Western Africa and Northern Africa. In Southern Africa, there are 5 countries: Botswana, Lesotho, Namibia, South Africa and Swaziland. Eastern Africa has 17 countries: Burundi, Comoros, Djibouti, Eritrea, Ethiopia, Kenya, Madagascar, Malawi, Mauritius, Mozambique, Rwanda, Seychelles, Somalia, Uganda, The United Republic of Tanzania, Zambia and Zimbabwe. In Middle Africa there are 9 countries: Angola, Cameroon, Central African Republic, Chad, Congo, Democratic Republic of the Congo, Equatorial Guinea, Gabon, Sao Tome and Principe. Western Africa is comprised of 16 countries: Benin, Burkina Faso, Cape Verde, Côte d'Ivoire, Gambia, Ghana, Guinea, Guinea-Bissau, Liberia, Mali, Mauritania, Niger, Nigeria, Senegal, Sierra Leone and Togo. There are 6 countries in Northern Africa: Algeria, Egypt, Libya Arab Jamahiriya, Morocco, Sudan and Tunisia.

African countries are not the same and yet they are the same. They are not the same in size and population. Some countries are more rural and some countries are more urban. Some countries are very poor with no national resources. Some countries are rich with natural resources like gold, diamonds, oil, rubber and coal. Some countries have never been colonized. They are African kingdoms that are still ruled by kings, for example, Swaziland. Other African countries have been colonized by different colonialists, for example, Britain colonized South Africa, France colonized Côte d'Ivoire, etc. Of 53 countries, 18 speak French, 18 speak English, 4 speak Arabic and French, and 3 speak Arabic and English, 5 Portuguese, 2 Spanish, 1 English and Swahili, 1 English and Amhara, and 1 French and English and indigenous languages. Some countries got their independence a long time ago, like Ghana that became independent in 1957, others like South Africa, have only received their independence recently, in the mid-nineties. Some countries had coup d'etat with military rule like Nigeria. Some won their independence through war, like Mozambique. Some countries are moving towards socialism, like Zimbabwe, and others to capitalism, like Botswana. Some countries are developing with strong economic growth, like Uganda (7.1%) and some are not, like Sierra Leone (-4.6%), according to the World Bank data.

South Africa is two countries in one. The African areas are not developed because of the legacy of Apartheid: whereas, the areas where the whites have lived are developed. The challenge for the government is to reconcile the two unequal worlds.

Each country has ethnic groups that speak different languages, for example, South Africa has 11 languages that are spoken such as Sepedi, Setswana, Seswazi, English, Afrikaans, Xhosa, Tshivenda, IsiZulu, IsiXhosa, IsiSwati and IsiNdebele. Nigeria has three languages, Ibo, Yoruba and Hausa. In Kenya there are more than four languages, Kikuyu,, Kamba, Luhya, Nyika and others. There are also countries with one ethnic group, for example, Botswana, Lesotho, Swaziland. Other countries also have one single language even though they may not be the same ethnic group, for example, Rwanda, Burundi, Somalia. In some countries, tribalism is strong, affecting the government and economy of the country.

Some countries have more Caucasians, like South Africa and Zimbabwe, and some have fewer Caucasians, like Nigeria. The Northern African countries are separated from other parts of Africa by the Sahara Desert, hence the term "Sub-Saharan Africa." Africa has different religions: African religions, Christianity, and Islam. Northern African countries and some of Western African countries practice Islam, for example, Libya and Mali. Many countries that have been colonized by Britain and France practice Christianity, for example, Malawi, Cameroon.

Even though there are differences, Africa is also the same. The African countries are undergoing similar problems: poverty, disease, low literacy, discrimination, exploitation by developed countries, human rights issues, difficult political transitions, lack of transparency in the government, centralized governments, refugee hosting and refugee generating. Most of the political leaders stay in power for a long time. Some are overthrown by coup d'etat. I salute President Nelson Mandela who broke the African political traditional role by serving only one term and then retiring. There are also some African countries, if they like their leaders, they like them to serve for a long time, like President Julius Nyerere of Tanzania. (I admired him. He was not greedy; he was a selfless and humble leader.)

Africa has similarities in solidarity during the struggle against colonialism and Apartheid. African countries helped freedom fighters from other countries that were still fighting for their liberation. They provided residence, passports, and they were advocates for freedom fighters through Organization of African Unity and through Non-Aligned Government Alliances and through The United Nations. When I fled South Africa in 1980 into Botswana, there were refugee camps for South Africans, Basothos, and Namibians. The Zimbabweans had just repatriated because they had gotten their independence. Zambia was the headquarters of the African National Congress. Our struggle against Apartheid was supported by Kenneth Kaunda's government. The same support was demonstrated in other African countries like Tanzania, Nigeria, and many others. These countries isolated apartheid-gripped South Africa and supported the liberation movements.

Polygamy is still the norm, as many women are still not educated and stay at home to raise children. Some women work as domestics, factory workers and farm laborers. Africa was once upon a time a cradle of civilization, rich with strong resilient people. Africa has gone through the tough times of colonialism, neo-colonialism and Apartheid, and has conquered those systems. I never thought that Apartheid would be abolished during my lifetime, but it was. There are challenges now in Africa, like military conflicts, forced internal displacement, refugee crises, poverty, poor housing, poor water supply, poor sanitation, illiteracy and diseases (AIDS, TB, malaria etc.). In most cases the rich keep getting richer and the poor keep getting poorer. It is estimated that 25 million out of the population of 778.4 million have died of AIDS. The challenge is to stop others from being infected with the HIV and to decrease the number of new cases. I believe with God in us, before and behind us, and beside us, we shall conquer HIV and AIDS. If we take personal responsibility, if families take their roles seriously, if non-governmental organizations give assistance, if governments promote stability, peace and development, if religious organizations, business and international organizations work together without blaming each other, exercising tolerance and unity on what we agree upon, Africa shall rise up in the 21st century and take her position in the world, where God wants her to be. There must be righteousness, justice, peace and prosperity. Without these, we will not be able to build an infrastructure and fight diseases including AIDS.

CHAPTER 2

The ABC of Viruses, HIV and AIDS

My people are destroyed from lack of knowledge (Hosea 4:6). They perish because of lack of knowledge, yet newspapers, television, internet and radio are filled with information about AIDS and HIV in Africa. There has been debate on whether HIV causes AIDS or not, and the president of South Africa, Dr. Thabo Mbeki was criticized for his analytic mind when he inquired whether HIV causes AIDS. Asking questions is never a bad move, since the more we inquire about facts, the more we learn. Our knowledge base increases, provided we get the correct information and not propaganda.

I cannot assume that everyone knows much about the viruses, especially HIV. If by any chance you know more about viruses and HIV, repetition is never a bad idea because it checks what you already know. In this chapter, I will simply explain, and not too technically, the concept of viruses: what are viruses, how do they get in our bodies, what happens when they are in our bodies, how can we prevent them from infecting us, and, briefly, how are they treated? Also, I will explain about the immune system, HIV and AIDS.

Susan Santag, the philosopher and critic, in *Illness as Metaphor* (Hilia) states, "Everyone who is born holds dual citizenship in the kingdom of the well and in the kingdom of the sick." Arthur Frank writes, "Illness takes away parts of your life, but in doing so it gives you the opportunity to choose the life you will lead as opposed to living out the one you have simply accumulated over the years."

There are many factors that cause diseases. Heredity is one factor, in which you get a disease because of the family genetic make-up (disease runs in your family). Aging is another factor which may lead to the development of diseases. As you grow older, your body activity slows down and your body structure degenerates and some diseases like arthritis, eye diseases and memory loss are created. The environment is also a predisposing factor for disease development, especially in Africa where, in most areas, there is still poor housing, poor sanitation, unclean water supply, mosquitoes and landmines. All this is exacerbated by poverty and conflict.

There are microorganisms that in other words are called "germs" that cause diseases. These are tiny organisms that cannot be seen by the naked eye. They can be seen by microscopes, however. Some microorganisms are good to our bodies and some cause infectious diseases. The microorganisms that are helpful are escherichia coli found in the digestive tract.

Pathogens are microorganisms that enter into the body and cause the diseases. Our bodies are created in such a way that if a pathogen enters, they will be able to protect themselves against the intruder or enemy. The body will use the physical, chemical and cellular forms to protect itself through the immune system. There are six harmful microorganisms, namely, viruses, bacteria, rickettsia, fungi, protozoa and parasitic worms. I will only discuss the viruses in this book.

What are viruses?

Viruses are the smallest and toughest pathogens. They are the toughest to fight because it is difficult to find drugs that will kill the virus without killing the host cells it has taken over. The virus cannot exist by itself. To be able to survive, and reproduce, it must attach itself to a host cell and inject its own DNA or RNA to trick the cell's reproductive functions into producing new viruses. Viruses cannot grow outside the cell. They are common; they are many. Some viruses are associated with common cold, influenza, mononucleosis, hepatitis, mumps, chicken pox, measles, rubella, polio and the human immuno deficiency virus that causes AIDS.

Viruses vary in their severity. Some viruses cause mild, short-lived illnesses for, example, flu for a day. Others are dangerous, causing hepatitis (inflammation of the liver), polio and AIDS. How do these small, toughest viruses get into our bodies? We are the hosts. How do we make it possible for them to enter? How do we get infected?

The virus must come into contact with a susceptible cell to invade it and to thrive. If it comes in contact with a dead cell, it cannot infect and grow, thus the skin becomes the protective layer as it is covered with dead cells that we wash daily. If your skin is broken by bites, a transfusion, or injections, then a virus like HIV or Hepatitis B, will be able to infect and grow in your body easily and cause AIDS or Hepatitis B.

Some viruses can be transported into the respiratory track through the air we breathe. These viruses can infect the nose, wind-pipe, bronchial tube and lungs and cause influenza and common cold. Other viruses can infect the digestive tract from the mouth, the esophagus, stomach, and intestines, and cause hepatitis A and various diarrheas. Viruses can also be carried through the anal and genital track during sexual intercourse. These viruses cause sexually transmitted diseases like AIDS.

In controlling the viral infection, it is important to understand and remember the types of viruses and the routes they take to enter one's body. To be able to prevent HIV, one must understand the route of transmission, which is through sexual intercourse through the anus or vagina and also through broken skin, transfusions of untested blood, use of HIV infected needles for injections and drug use, and from the HIV infected pregnant mother to the fetus.

What happens when the virus infects?

In an experiment in the laboratory where a purified virus preparation is used to infect cells, the viral infection cycle is divided into several events, according to Hung Fan, et al.

First, the virus binds to the cell. The viral particle interacts with some protein on the surface of the cell. This protein is the virus receptor. At this period, absorption or binding takes place. While the viral particle is attached to the receptor protein, the second phase takes place, in which the virus penetrates the cell. When it gets into the cell, the virus removes its protective coat, thus exposing its genetic material. This period in the cycle is called penetration. The uncoated virus cannot withstand the condition in the cell and that accounts for a drop in infection. Thirdly, when the infectious virus in the culture is low, during the eclipse period, several things happen: the expression of the virus genes, which may lead to the death of the infected cell: production of the viral genetic material; and the production of the proteins for viral particles for the virus coat and the envelope within the infected cell. Fourthly, there is an assembly of new infectious viruses, and they are released from the cells, and the amount of infectious virus is more than at the beginning of the infection.

In the human body, there is an immune system that responds to the spread of virus particles to infect other cells, depending on whether the virus is lytic, non lytic or latent. When the infected cell is killed at the end of infection, the virus is called lytic. The virus is non lytic when the infected cells are not killed at the end of infection, but form a persistent or carrier state.

In some cases, viruses can remain hidden in the cell and do not produce other viruses. They can be in a state of latency. These are latent viruses. They may be reactivated and produce infectious virus particles at a later time.

How do we treat the viral infection?

Viruses are difficult to treat. By comparison, bacteria can be effectively treated by antibiotics, because they block the intracellular (inside the cell) machinery used to make proteins in bacteria and not in humans. However, in viral infection, it is difficult to find drugs that are the same as antibiotics, that will block the growth of viruses in the cells without killing the infected cell, because viruses rely on the cell to carry its breaking and building up process.

There are few cases where viral infections can be blocked by antiretroviral drugs. Medications such as Azidothymidine (Zidovudine) or AZT can inhibit the human immuno deficiency virus (HIV). Viral vaccines are also used before the individual is infected with the virus. Most viral infections today are controlled by treating the symptoms—fever (aspirin), secondary infections (classic antibiotics), and fatigue (bed rest).

The treatment of viruses is difficult because of their nature, how they invade the human cell, the cycle they go through, absorption, penetration and uncoating of genetic materials, expression of the viral genetic material and its assembly inside the infected cell and its release from the cell to infect the other cells. Antiretroviral drugs do not destroy the virus. Therefore, the best management of the viral infection especially HIV is to prevent the first infection. Human immuno deficiency virus, HIV is preventable.

The immune system

Let me now explore the process of infection and how our body responds through the immune system, our defense system against invasion by the enemies, which can be bacteria, viruses, protozoa and fungi. The immune system is the system that protects the body from infection by foreign bodies or micro-organisms. The defense system has different types of "soldiers," trained to fight a specific invader, in a specific way. The immune system is made of two types of cells: the lymphocytes and the phagocytes. The lymphocytes attack the specific foreign agent and the phagocytes attack and eat that foreign agent. Phagein is a Greek word meaning "to eat." Phagocytes are further divided into two: the macrophages and the neutrophils. The macrophages, located in blood and tissues, attack and eat cells infected with viruses (foreign agents). The neutrophils attack bacteria. Mast cells, basophils and eosinophils attack bigger infectious agents. They release the toxic (poisonous) substance that kills foreign agents.

In the immune system, there are lymphocytes that respond to a specific foreign agent. There are two types of lymphocytes. The B cells and the T cells. The B cells produce the antibodies that bind directly and neutralize the work of the infectious agent. The T cells are divided into two types: the T helper cells and the T killer cells. The T helper cells do not kill cells carrying the infectious agent. They interact with the B cells and the T killer cells and help to respond to the infectious agent (antigen). The T killer cells directly bind to the cells that carry the infectious agent and kill them. The T killer and the T helper cells each have proteins on their surfaces. On the surface of the T killer cells, there is CD8 protein, and on the T helper cells, CD4 protein. There are tests that have been made to identify the count of the T helper and the T killer cells.

In a normal functioning immune system, when an infectious agent gets into the body, the eating cells (phagocytes) confront the enemy and attempt to engulf it and eat it. The macrophages call the T helper cells to the scene. The T helper cells identify the infectious agent and call the T killer cells to destroy the infectious agent. Also, the T helper cells call the B cells to produce the antibodies to attack and destroy the infectious agent. At the end of the fight, the memory cells are activated, giving the body immunity following the attack. Suppressor T cells come to the scene after the battle is won to suppress the production of antibodies.

The process is incredible. If you did not understand it clearly because of these technical words, I will explain it in a simpler way. When you are residing in a village or township with roads going in and out, that village or township will want to protect itself against enemies. What will happen is, the leaders of the village or township will place some people at the entrances to spot enemies. If they see enemies, they will have certain sounds to tell the soldiers to come and attack these enemies. The soldiers will come, already armed with the correct ammunitions, to the correct areas and attack the enemy and defend the village or the township. The T helper cells help by calling the T killer cells and B cells to attack the enemy. In most cases, the battle is won. In the case of the HIV, the virus attacks the T helper cells, the important cells that give signs or alarms to the attackers (T killer cells and B cells). If these T helper cells are attacked, they are not able to call the strong army, the T killer cells and B cells. Hence the defense is not warned, and the HIV attacks the body. Thus the whole village or township will be invaded and attacked by enemies because the species (T helper cells) are paralyzed. The village becomes defenseless and deficient. That is why the virus is called human deficiency virus, because it makes the immune system deficient, not adequate in performing its task of attacking the virus.

What is HIV?

Human Immunodeficiency Virus is a retrovirus. The genetic information of the retrovirus is RNA that is covered with a viral protein coat to make the core particle. The core particle is covered with a viral envelope that contains fats and viral proteins. The characteristics of the retrovirus are: First, they do not kill cells; they invade. They can form a stable carrier state within the infected cell because they integrate their DNA into the person's infected chromosomes. When an opportunity comes for infection, the virus will be activated. The enzyme reverse transcriptionase comes out the process of converting the virus RNA genetic information into DNA. This is why these viruses are called retroviruses, because they reverse the flow of genetic information.

Human Immunodeficiency Virus, HIV, is also a lenti virus in the family of the retrovirus. The lenti viruses are slow viruses and the spread of the disease is also slow. That is why HIV takes a long time to be detected and produce the signs and symptoms.

There are other names that have been used for HIV. They are HTIV-III, LAV and ARV. The HIV virus is dangerous, because when it infects the cells, it kills the T helper lymphocytes that are the important gatekeeper cells for the immune system. Also the HIV infects the macrophages (eating cells) that are the front line defenders of the body against the invaders. Unlike in the T helper cells, which kill HIV, the HIV virus does not kill the macrophages (eating cells). Some of these eating cells continue to produce HIV viruses while the others form the latent state of the HIV infection. They form a reservoir of infection in a person who is HIV infected.

The Human Immunodeficiency Virus attacks the body's defense system and makes it deficient, not able to protect the body against the enemy. That is why, in the fight against AIDS, understanding how the HIV works is crucial, so that we can do everything possible in our power to keep the HIV outside the human body.

Human Immunodeficiency Virus is an opportunistic virus. That means, whenever and however it gets an opportunity to enter the human, it will. The HIV does not discriminate. It makes no difference whether you are Black or White, whether you are rich or poor, whether you are educated or non educated, whether you live in the urban city or rural area, whether you are religious or irreligious, whether you are male or female, whether you are young or old. If an individual is involved in high risk behavior with someone infected, that gives the HIV the opportunity to infect the body.

The HIV infection will eventually lead to Acquired immunedeficiency syndrome (AIDS). Acquired means that the person was not born with the disease, but he or she got it from somewhere, in this case, from someone infected with HIV. Immune deficiency means that the individual's immune system is no longer effective in fighting the infection because the HIV has crippled the soldier T helper cells that alarm the heavy army, T killer and B cells to fight. The body, therefore, is unable to fight infections. Syndrome means a group of different signs and symptoms that are associated with the disease.

When a person is infected with the HIV virus, he or she does not develop AIDS the following day, but there is a journey that begins and it unfolds itself in different ways. First, when the HIV has infected an individual it takes a slow progression. Remember that HIV is a lentivirus, it spreads the disease slowly, affecting the immune system. It can take an average of 10 years before the signs and symptoms show up. Sometimes it can take fewer years depending on the socio-economic and physical condition of an individual.

Even though not everyone who has been exposed to HIV gets AIDS, it is important to keep the HIV outside the human body. Human immuno deficiency virus is preventable. HIV can be found in body fluids of infected people, in vaginal secretions, semen, blood, and breast milk. The body fluids that hardly ever contain little live cells of HIV are saliva, tears, perspiration, urine and feces.

HIV testing

The HIV Antibody Test has been developed to test whether the individual has been exposed to the virus by checking if the person has antibodies to the HIV proteins. Infected persons begin to produce HIV antibodies (seroconvert) 2 to 3 months after exposure. This is variable, as the window period can last for a year. There are two HIV antibody tests that are used. They are ELIZA and Western Blot. The current ELIZA is 99.9% accurate. Western Blot is used to confirm the results of ELIZA because it has lower false positives than ELIZA. False positive means the test will read positive when you are negative. False negative appears when an individual is infected and the test shows negative. More follow up tests must be done at different times. There are some tests that are more sensitive for HIV, testing the virus particles. These are based on a technique called polymerase chain reaction or PCR.

It is important for individuals to have pre-counseling before the test and post-counseling after the test. The results of the tests are confidential. There are ethical questions around HIV testing. People should not be coerced to take HIV tests. Also, there are moral questions about HIV, such as whether people should be screened when there is no adequate treatment. Individuals can be HIV positive and infectious but not have signs and symptoms.

Diagnosis of AIDS

When an HIV infected person develops physical symptoms he is diagnosed with AIDS. Factors that influence physical symptoms are sex, age, genetic makeup, nutrition, environmental factors and encounters with other infectious diseases.

The initial symptoms of AIDS are wasting syndrome, loss of body weight, fevers at night, night sweats, diarrhea, high temperature. There may be swelling of the lymph glands called lymphadenopathy syndrome (LAS). Swelling of the lymph glands in the head, neck, armpits and the groin. If the swelling persists, it is called the persistent generalized lymphadenopathy (PGL). There are also psychological and neurological diseases like dementia (inability to remember), depression, social withdrawal and personality changes. Spinal cord damage (myelopathy) which may end up with weakness and paralysis of voluntary muscles and peripheral nerve damage (neuropathy) can also occur. Different people develop different symptoms.

When the immune system is damaged, infections occur, for example, Candida, a fungal infection. There is also thrush and could be esophagitis (inflammation of the esophagus) and hairy leukoplakia (white plagues on the surface of the tongue and the esophagus).

The full-blown AIDS has opportunistic infections such as inflammation of the lungs (Pneumocytis carinii Pneumonia PCP), Inflammation of intestinal tract (Cryptosporidium gastroenterritis), cancers, (Kaposi sarcoma) Tuberculosis, lymphomas and cervical cancers, to name a few. There is no one treatment for AIDS. Various physical symptoms are managed according to the opportunistic infections that prevail.

Unfortunately, no one has been healed from this disease. Some people live longer with the HIV and do not progress to AIDS. Others who have AIDS can receive the antiretroviral drugs that will treat the symptoms and slow the progression to full-blown AIDS and prolong life but will not cure the disease. For detailed AIDS statistics, see Appendix A.

CHAPTER 3

Human Immune Deficiency Virus Is Preventable

I have been part of the HIV/AIDS education curriculum development process since 1986, and I am convinced that the critical issues about HIV/AIDS are proper information, education and knowledge about the Human Immune Deficiency Virus, and a change of attitude and behavior. There is still misinformation about HIV, what it is, and what the virus can and cannot do in the human body or outside the human body. Most people feel hopeless about HIV/AIDS, as if nothing can be done by individuals to stop the HIV infection. In this chapter, I will discuss that HIV is preventable, provided we are going to ask the simple question, "Do I want to die or live?" If your decision is to live, then you must radically change your attitude and behavior towards what makes the HIV easy to enter your body.

Now we know that there are three "doors" in which the HIV enters into the human body. The first "door" that is most frequently used is the sexual transmission. The second "door" is the intravenous transmission through HIV infected blood transfusion and drug use. The third "door" is the HIV infected pregnant mother to child transmission, where an infected mother infects the unborn baby during pregnancy and, after birth, during breastfeeding.

What an individual can do must be determined, motivated and inspired by his or her vision that he or she can be a victor and not a victim of HIV. The determination to life is the first step in fighting to keep the HIV outside your body. Now that you have chosen life, you need, first, to revolutionize your sexual outlook and behavior.

Sexual intercourse is a gift of God to human beings to express their affection to each other, and to procreate, to have children. One of my teachers in high school in South Africa used to emphasize to us that sex is good with the right person, at the right time and in the right place. He said the right person was your husband or wife, the right time was when you are married and the right place was your home. This was the sex education he gave to us. He emphasized the virtue of waiting until the right person comes along at the right time and in the right place.

He was trying to combine sex education with values.

Did we all wait until we met the right person, at the right time, in our home? Some did, some did not. However, even if you did not wait, you knew that was the right thing to do. There were certain consequences which some who didn't wait experienced: teenage pregnancy, sexually transmitted diseases, not being able to complete their education. These consequences often led to work in low paying jobs and poverty.

Today, sexual intercourse puts people at high risk for premature death through HIV infection. Most young people are experimenting with sex, and that is a "gun loaded with bullets" because HIV is not written on the face of individuals. Also, people are not honest with their sexual histories if they are asked.

What should young people and single people do to stop the HIV from entering their body sexually? The answer is: abstinence or postponement of sexual intercourse.

I can hear you saying, "That is not possible. It cannot happen. Sex is natural." I understand that response. That is a natural reaction. I heard it before and I still hear it now. Yes, sex is natural, but we can, nevertheless, exercise self control. I still say that abstinence is the perfect way (100%) to prevent HIV sexual transmission and it is possible, with the help of others, if your choice is life and not death. Abstinence from sex may be difficult, but, in the absence of vaccine and medicine to cure the disease, affordable drugs, the capacity to administer the drugs even if they're free, it's something one must consider seriously. It may be a difficult road to travel but it is not an impossible road to travel if you have encouragement, help and resources along the way.

How do we help young people to abstain from sex? Do we only say "say no to sex" or are we engaging them in issues and programs that are empowering and affirming their destiny as future leaders and productive citizens of their country? First, we have to convince ourselves, and the young people, that they can postpone sexual intercourse. They must, because they have a lot to offer in this world, and the HIV should not be cutting short that destiny.

Sex education should be taught within the political, cultural and spiritual context of Africa. Young people should be taught that Africa was under the colonial ruler and there were some Africans who dedicated their lives to liberating Africa. To some, it was an impossibility, but those who had the "war spirit" in their hearts about freedom, fought in the liberation struggles and all African countries are now politically free.

On June 16, 1976, in South Africa, we were the young people who demonstrated against Apartheid. The demonstration began as a protest against the imposition of Afrikaans (the oppressor's language) as a medium of instruction in schools. We had the power, zeal and determination to stand up against Apartheid and the military power. We had a political purpose. Our struggle echoed internationally. Now that we have political freedom, the young people of today should be involved in the transformation and development of the country, and HIV should not stand in the way of fulfilling those dreams.

We are at war now with HIV and we need that "war spirit" to fight HIV and AIDS. We need that spirit of "de-revolutionizing sex" by young people. This begins with the young men and how they view young women. Young women have a lot to offer as well as young men. Young men should respect young women, and young women should respect young men. Young people can be happy and enjoy the company of each other with respect and without having sex.

In 1987, I gave a talk on HIV/AIDS to high school students in Baltimore, Maryland. I discussed with them the ABC's of HIV and how to prevent HIV. I emphasized that the best way to prevent HIV was to abstain from sex until you marry because you will be able to reach your educational goals without pregnancy and possible HIV infection. One student asked, "What is abstinence?" She had never heard the word before. I replied, "Not having sex with your boyfriend." To my surprise I did not encounter resistance from them. They liked the linkage of HIV prevention with their educational goals in future. One student came to me after the class and thanked me for saying that. She said, "I wish my parents could tell me so that I can know and do that."

What I learned was that young people are not impressed by the defeatist attitude that adults have that they cannot abstain. In fact they are receptive to the idea that they can postpone sex with resources provided in empowerment and leadership programs.

The attitude that everything is surrounded by sex and no one can do anything about it, should be replaced by a new attitude: Everything is not surrounded by sex but by the individual's mind and spirit, striving to reach his or her destiny in life.

In order to remove the barriers that make abstinence an impossible task, we have to stop glamorizing high-risk behaviors, for example prostitution. I know we have a fancy name for it, commercial sex workers. But prostitution is an exploitation of women and in some cases men. Prostitution takes advantage of poor women who are not educated. The only time they can sleep in a fancy hotel is when a rich man brings them there to have sex with them for a fee. In most cases, their fee is less than that of the escort business owner who arranges the meetings.

The destiny of African young girls is not prostitution, but to be teachers, nurses, medical doctors, prophets, priests, engineers, scientists, politicians, economists, physicians and farmers. And the list goes on. They must be trained so that they can be involved in professions that are currently underrepresented by women in their countries. Certainly African women are capable of using their heads, hearts and hands and not necessarily their sexual organs.

As an African mother, I would like my son and daughter to succeed in the world, to make a productive impact in the development of the country but not in prostitution. If we love our young people, we shall put values in their heads and hearts to follow and succeed in life. Chastity and character education clubs should be a part of HIV prevention programs. They should be funded so that young people can be motivated to stay abstinent. Young people need incentives and encouragement. They need to hear such messages from elders they trust and respect. They are our princes and princesses, not our prostitutes. They should be taught about how to create a positive relationship and how to drop it when it is abusive. They must be advised about how far to go in dating. Parents and health educators should keep teaching the idea that the young people can be saved from HIV if they stop having sex before and outside of marriage. In

Baltimore where I live, there are billboards that proclaim: "Virgin is not a dirty word. Teach your children." These are the words to be taught to our young people. Songs should be written and performed on abstinence from sex. I read that, in Mozambique, abstinence is not working, because the young girls get married to older men who infect them with HIV. The problem there is not abstinence but the infidelity of older men. Adultery puts everyone at risk. Abstinence is not only a virtue for girls and women, but also for boys and men.

Married couples must take responsibility for protecting each other. The monogamous sexual relationship is very important. If one needs to live, one should remove the attitude that sleeping around with many women when you are married makes you a better and more powerful man. A good, strong, powerful man is the one who respects his wife and does not humiliate her by sleeping around with other women. I am aware of the polygamous marriage and that will be dealt with in Chapter 4.

What should a person do to prevent HIV if that person does not abstain from sex? Use condoms. These are thin, tight-fitting sheaths of latex rubber or animal skin. Latex rubber condoms are preferable. Some condoms are coated with spermicides like nonoxynol-9. These condoms are effective in killing sperms. Do not use Vaseline and other oil to lubricate the condom. When you have decided to use condoms, make sure that when you buy them, you check the expiration date. Do not store them in places that have heat that can cause the rubber to deteriorate. Do not reuse a condom.

There are still risks in using the condom. It may break, as it is rubber. It may slip out. In the use of condoms, there is also a problem of access, distribution and utilization. Can everyone who needs a condom in Africa get one? Does that person have money to buy condoms? Where I am, a condom costs US$1:00 per condom. US$1:00 is equivalent to R7 or R8 South African money. Can condoms be distributed to the remote villages? Condom use is unnatural and most Africans resist using them. But even though the idea of condom use is foreign, there are many African men who want to live. So, when it's a choice between abstaining from sex and having sex using condoms, they chose the latter.

African women who have decided to have sex, must be taught negotiation skills to ask the men to use condoms. When one has decided to use a condom and have sex, one should limit the anal sex as it is highly risky. The rectum is part of the digestive system. It is the exit for food that was not used by the body. It is not an entrance for sexual intercourse. CONDOMS ARE GOOD; ABSTINENCE IS BEST.

God created sex. It is when we step outside the discipline of God that we fall into trouble. We are not animals, discipline and self- control are important and an individual should make that decision out of the values he or she was raised with in the home. The individual will understand that he or she is above the animal kingdom. Self-control is best for him or her. If one takes the first step, then God, family, community will assist in taking the rest. There will be negative forces that will say that abstinence is not possible. Yes, self-control is possible. Just try it. It is safe and cheap.

CHAPTER 4

The Role of the African Family

The African family does not have boundaries. The African family is not the nuclear family. Mother and father are not the only parents, but mother's sisters and brothers and father's brothers and sisters. In the African family, your mother's sisters are your mothers. Whether they are older or younger than your mother. In Sesotho, Setswana, Sepedi, isiZulu, and isiXhosa the elder sisters of your mother are called mmamoholo, mamogolo umamkhulu where "mma" means mother and "holo" or "golo" "mkhulu" means senior. The younger sisters of your mother are called mmangwane, mmane, umamuncane where "mma" means mother and "ngwane", "mane" "mcane" means junior. You have your mother, senior and junior mothers. You do not have one mother in the African culture.

The same is true for the father. The brothers of your father are your fathers. In Sesotho, Setswana, Sepedi, isiZulu, the elder brothers of the father are ntatemoholo, rremogolo, ramogolo, babamkhulu where ntate, nre, ra, baba mean father and moholo, mogolo, mkhulu mean senior. The junior brothers of the father are rangwane, babamcane where ngwane, mcane mean junior. You have senior fathers and junior fathers. The brother to the mother is malome, uncle, and this uncle has a critical role in the upbringing of his sister's children. "ditlogolo, isizukulu" niece and nephews. They all have a single word, no feminine or masculine version. The father's sisters also play a critical role in raising her brother's children. She is called Rakgadi, "ra" means father and "kgadi" female, the father's sister. Everyone is a family member. The grandparents are also parents taking care of grandchildren. They are not put into an institution.

In most African countries, polygamy was and still is the dominant force in marriage. My maternal grandfather's brother married more than one wife. They are my grandmothers. My maternal grandfather was converted to Christianity and went to school. He married one wife, my grandmother. I grew up with many grandparents, senior and junior mothers from maternal and paternal families. Most families were like that.

Some polygamous marriages were formed because the first wife was barren. Africans revered children, that is why, in most African countries, abortion is hard to sell. Some first wives are involved in picking the second or third or more wives. In polygamous marriages, families are larger. In African countries that practice Islam religion, the families have also more than one wife, and the family is big.

As Africans moved from the rural areas to urban areas, some became educated and converted to Christianity, and became monogamous, but they still have strong African family ties. The orphans did not have a problem, as their senior or junior fathers, senior or junior mothers, uncles, aunts looked after them. My mother was the youngest of the five daughters of my grandmother and grandfather. Her older sister, No. 2, died and her husband died. They had two children who were then raised by my mother and her elder sister. When my mother was very ill, her sisters took care of me and the others. Later, when all her sisters died, mother was able to look after their children. All the children were considered my brothers and sisters.

When I visited the rural areas and other countries, Botswana, Zambia, Nigeria, I also observed strong family ties, strong marriages and large families. These African family ties and marriages were made strong by the foundation on which they were formed. When a young man was to marry a young girl, it was not the decision of the two only. Rather, both families met, slaughtered cattle or sheep, and negotiated "lobola" the bridal price. In their culture they were not buying a wife, but saying thank you to the girl's family. Big weddings were planned and took a week to a month depending on the distances between the bride and groom. The whole village celebrated the wedding.

Urbanization, colonization, Apartheid and political wars have affected the African family. In South Africa, fathers were separated from their families to work in the mines. They were living in unlivable hostels and were allowed to go home once a year, during Christmas and New Year's time. Some were not able to go back. Migratory labor was from Malawi, Zimbabwe, Mozambique, Botswana, Lesotho, Swaziland. They married women in the city who also came to work as domestic servants or factory workers. In Soweto where I grew up, there were different ethnic groups. There were intermarriages within tribes, and families ties were still strong.

Every country in Africa was colonized by different colonizers— French, British, Portuguese—at different times, and the struggle to fight colonialism took many forms that affected the African family. However, colonialism and Apartheid were not only the ills that affected the African family. The destabilization of free African countries that ended with coup d'etat and wars, also affected the African family.

I was invited to participate in the conflict resolution conference for women in Liberia before general elections. We listened and cried together as the women were relating the atrocities which happened to them, especially rapes. One wondered what had happened to the African family where women were treated as queens, daughters as princesses? What had happened to the time when African kings, chiefs and older men could come to the castle and solve the problems of the community without sending the army on their own people? We still have a few countries in Africa that never waged war on their citizens.

We need to ask these questions: After the African family has gone through changes, does it still have a role in preventing HIV and caring for family members suffering from AIDS? If it does, what should the African family do to minimize the HIV infection and care for persons with AIDS and their orphans?

First, we have to go back to the position in African family culture of respecting girls and women. They need to be empowered, as they are home and community builders. I still remember the time when a father, his brothers and the mother's brothers would not hurt a baby girl because it was their baby. You trusted your fathers and uncles, knowing that they would respect you and not harm you. Raping children was unthinkable and shameful.

Secondly, African men must protect the African family. When African families were invaded by enemies in the past, African men protected them. Today, African men cannot afford to expose their daughters and wives to danger. The spiritual and social consciousness of looking at all girls as daughters and all women, especially wives as queens, needs to be revived. They need to respect their women, not force them to do what they are not ready to do.

Thirdly, the men should be monogamous, have one wife. Adultery is a risky business. Men should also abstain from sex; if they can't, they should use condoms. Protection should not be the burden of women only. Men in polygamous marriages need to be faithful to those wives. I am for one husband, one wife, but I cannot tell the polygamous husbands to divorce their wives. However, they can protect them from HIV by being responsible and faithful. As the society changes and more women and men are educated and become influenced by socioeconomic and spiritual factors, polygamy will fade away. It is already happening. More people are marrying only one wife, though some still have mistresses, who pose a risk for HIV/AIDS.

The African men must provide for the African family. I do understand that unemployment is rising in African countries. (This problem will be dealt in Chapters 7 and 8 when we deal with the role of government and industry.) Nevertheless, sons and daughters should be raised to take leadership in the society.

African mothers must also respect African fathers. I am aware that these days, there are concepts like feminism, where women fight domination by men and womanism where African women fight domination by race and men. I may consider myself a womanist, but I have learned not to fight the men, but, rather, the system. Patriarchy and racism should not be fought only by women, but also by men. African sisterhood is paramount. Hence, "sisters" should stay away from the husbands of their "sisters." We must instill in our young girls that they are not inferior beings because they are females. They are strong and they can become powerful because they are made in the image of God.

Sex is not always something about which people can talk. I learned that girls and boys who went to mountains in the winter to be circumcised were taught about male and female relationships and sex. I was always curious to know the details of what happened, but I was told it was secret, and, if I wanted to know, I should go. My family was Christian and we were not allowed to go.

Some African countries still practice female circumcision, which harmful to young girls. This is one of the African cultural ideas which needs to be revamped, especially in the light of HIV and AIDS. When they do a clitoridectomy (removal of the clitoris), blood is involved. Thus, circumcision is not safe, as it involves incisions and contact with blood.

What kind of sex education did we get in our family? How did we get it from our mothers? The sex education we received when we were little girls was that we should not do IT. We were told that a child comes in an airplane. My elder sister delivered her baby at home. I saw a nurse midwife come to the house, and I was told to go and play at the playground. When I came back, I found a baby girl. I asked my mother, "How did the baby come?" I had not seen any airplane. I was told the nurse went to the airplane and brought the baby in the suitcase. I was satisfied because I saw the nurse with the suitcase. Now I know it held the delivery apparatus. Most women delivered their babies at home. A few complicated deliveries were done in the hospital.

When a girl has her first menstrual period, a bit more sex education will be given. They will tell her not to sleep with a man because she will have a baby. She will either believe her mother and not sleep with a man or she will listen to friends, who challenge her mother's theory and tell her it is not really true, and urge her to experiment. Always after the experiment, whether it is once or twice or more, a young woman becomes pregnant and finds out that mother, with her simple sex education, "Don't sleep with a man you will be pregnant," was right. But it is too late. At school, some of us were fortunate to take biology and do nursing. This taught us to understand the anatomy and physiology of the body, how the body is made, how it functions, and especially how the reproductive organs function.

I am aware that many people in the villages, even in the urban areas, are not talking to their children about sex because they do not know in detail what to say. However, even in the old times, women had the insight to warn their children about sleeping around with men. In my community, a girl who slept around with many different men was named a "rubber neck" and people would look down upon her. It helped us as young girls, because we did not like that name. It helped us to be careful in our sexual behaviors. There was a double standard. The men were sanctioned to sleep around because we were told that they were dogs. It was okay for them. We read that in the Bible that when some men brought a woman to Jesus Christ because she was caught in adultery, the men she was caught with were not brought along. Who knows? The men who brought her might have been the ones, but the Bible did not record that. However, we knew Jesus' response, which gave us a hint of who might have been involved with this woman (John 8:3-11). In the prevention of HIV and AIDS we cannot afford a double social standard because everyone can be infected and everyone will eventually die since there is no cure.

In the prevention of HIV, we need those African values that inspire you to become good respected women and men affirmed by your family and the community. Men and women are needed who can be mentors of little boys and girls. The strength of the African family lies in the stability and resources of the country and also in holding onto the parts of African culture and values that make us strong people. We must forsake the parts of African culture and behaviors that demean women, like female circumcision, polygamy and prostitution.

Polygamy was good in past cultures, as men were few and women were many. It allowed single women to marry and bear children, and it allowed for a second wife, if the first wife was barren. But now that times have changed and men don't have the resources to support many women, polygamy needs to be revisited. I am proposing a different direction for the coming generation. With the spread of HIV, one man can infect all his wives, or one wife can infect the husband and other wives.

The African extended family has helped the orphans for many years and I believe we can use that positive culture to take care of AIDS orphans. I understand that lack of food, financial resources and lack of knowledge are the main causes why children are abandoned. More education for grandparents and resources for them will create a stable family in long term. I am concerned about institutionalizing children with AIDS in orphanages for a long time. It separates and stigmatizes them. The majority of orphanages around the world tend to have abuses in the long run.

The African family can trust in God, who during hard times, quickened their spirit. My family had rules, and one of them was to pray and to go to church to worship. They believed that God is the one who, when all have failed, will make us victors. In the village, the African family was close to God's creation, the trees, the rivers, the mountains, the valleys and they believed that there was One who rules this creation. Rev. Addo from Ghana, a man who walked with Kwame Nkrumah, says the African family will be saved when the family realizes that Jesus Christ, who has been hidden from Africa for political and economic reasons, is recognized. He came so that all people can understand that they are made in God's image and they can be saved.

CHAPTER 5

The Role of the African Non-Governmental Organization

Individuals and families may not have a strong impact without the help of non-governmental organizations (NGOs). In most cases these organizations are driven by need and passion on an issue. They organize around it. Some non-governmental organizations are pro their governments and some are not, especially those fighting for human rights. I remember during Apartheid, there were non-governmental organizations opposing the government. Even now, in other African countries led by governments that are not democratic, there is no cooperation between the governments and NGOs. In those countries NGOs face difficult times; they may be banned from operating or operate under difficult terms.

With the HIV-AIDS epidemic, there are some individual political rights which need to be challenged. When a person with HIV or AIDS is not allowed to be admitted to school, to work, to have privacy, NGOs become relevant in advocating those issues. Some African NGOs are humanitarian, assisting in delivery of services, and some are political. Most political NGOs tend to be on the left of the political spectrum. However with HIV & AIDS, NGOs will be shaped by the goal to prevent the spread of HIV and care for those who have AIDS rather than by political ideology. HIV does not discriminate between a leftwing person or a rightwing person. Human beings have to be smarter than the virus and work together.

Some new NGOs have a tough time establishing their legitimacy and credibility. I attended a meeting, a dialogue between African NGOs and American NGOs. One of the American NGOs raised a question to the group, "Who speaks for Africa." The question challenges the African NGOs to make sure they represent Africans. Are these mushrooming NGOs on AIDS speaking for Africa or have some NGOs been created to provide jobs for a few individuals? Are the funds being spent on overheads, project directors or services? (The question was not answered.) In the attempt to answer the question, "Who speaks for Africa?" African NGOs will need to establish a community involvement approach. Perhaps, the project could be owned by the community, rather than by a few smart people who know how to write proposals or grants and get funding. Better African NGOs are those that operate from Africa and are run by Africans and also by persons with HIV or AIDS. When African NGOs operates that way, there will not be any need to question who speaks for Africa, because the works of the African NGOs will speak for themselves.

There are two principles African non-governmental organizations need to be aware of. First, African non-governmental organizations should not be motivated by the source of funding but by the needs of the people they serve. When funding dictates or changes the core needs of the community, it results in the loss of money and the cause. I know that projects work even if there is not enough money because people do sacrifice for what they are passionate about. I also do not say that funding is not necessary, because it is.

The second principle is, to avoid competition that ends up in a duplication of services. In a village or township, there should not be several non-governmental organizations working against each other. This point will be further discussed under collaboration as methodology for NGOs.

Presently there are questions and misinformation about HIV and AIDS. One lady from Zimbabwe asked me, "How can we convince people in the village to use condoms?" One governmental official from Ethiopia in one of the meetings told us that it was difficult to convince people to use condoms because there is misinformation about the spermicide nonoxynol-9 that is applied at the tip of the condom. People were suspicious that that might be the virus, HIV.

Most pregnant African women do not want to be screened for HIV because they do not want to know and they cannot handle the news of being positive. One of the Motswana pregnant women said on the Maryland Public Television documentary on AIDS in Africa, that if she knew that she had the virus, she would kill herself. There are stories from family and friends in South Africa that there is a belief that having sex with the virgin will heal the HIV infection and AIDS. Hence, some men raped young girls thinking that they would be healed. All of these stories show how many different approaches are needed by different NGOs to prevent the HIV virus from spreading and to care for persons with AIDS.

I have a "three C's" approach to discuss which I believe the African non-governmental organizations can adopt to make education, the delivery of services, and clinical care easier and effective.

The first "C" is cultural sensitivity. I remember when I was a student in one of my public health courses at Johns Hopkins University, one of the professors told us this story in which public health professionals dealing with environmental health went to a country in Asia and found that there was a problem of poor sanitation in a village. They concluded that people needed latrines. They did not consult with the community, however. What they did was to look for grants, write a proposal, and they were awarded funding to build latrines. They had a time line that said, at the end of that the year, they should build about 50 or more latrines. They met their deadline, and when it was time for people to use the latrines, the people did not use the latrines. It was not in their culture to go into a small house for urination or defecation. The lesson was, whatever project you would like to do, you must discuss it with the community and be culturally sensitive, otherwise, it will not work. It does not matter what good intentions one might have, if it is condescending and patronizing, it will not work.

When I listen to the concerns of a woman from Zimbabwe, a government official from Ethiopia and the responses of a Motswana pregnant woman and myths about sex with the virgins, these tell me that we might be following an AIDS education script from America or Europe that is designed in a different culture other than African. We talk more about sex education in homes, schools or in the community, which I don't have a problem with if the curriculum is within the context of positive African culture. In going to give a presentation on HIV and AIDS in a village or township, you need to know the language and what should be in the presentation. Is it the goal to prevent HIV infection or do you have other political motives? If the goal is to make people aware of the disease and how they can prevent HIV infection, then explore with them what and how they can prevent HIV, before imposing condom use. In the first place, a condom is a rubber. It has sticky substance (spermicide) on the tip. It is a foreign body. I can understand why people do not want to use it. I thought of my extended family in the rural areas and of how I could convince them to use condoms. I asked myself some questions first. Are condoms the only way to prevent HIV infection? Are there other ways that are culturally accepted? Would it be easier to talk about African culture, where you were encouraged not to have sex until marriage first, rather than to convince them to use condoms? They can always be introduced to condom use, later, if it's necessary, when they're comfortable with the idea?

Even in the cities and townships we had those cultural values where you were shunned if you had a child outside of wedlock. In some cases girls who had babies and were not married to their children's fathers had a hard time getting married. Most African men are macho, they think because they paid "lobola" (dowry) a woman belongs to them. When they want to have sex, a woman must comply. She doesn't have the right to say no. In a polygamous marriage, all women must comply. Most men say they want to have sex without a condom. Would it not be easier to work with them on their role as protector of the family to protect their wives, sons and daughters from a HIV infection through self-control and empowerment in relationships as well as introducing the subject of condoms?

Yes, I understand that some cultural values are outdated and must be changed, like the one in Zimbabwe where the father-in-law has to have sex with the daughter-in-law before her husband after marriage. We should stand against them. Cultural sensitivity is important because changing behavior takes a long time. Being a modern person does not mean you have to be immoral sexually, especially in the era of HIV infection and AIDS. Sexual revolution needs a de-revolution. I believe we can dig deeper into all our African culture and find positive African mores that will help us to prevent the HIV infection. NGOs that are dealing with HIV prevention through education need to explore cultural sensitivity in their curricula.

The second "C" is collaboration. The strength of fighting the infection of HIV and AIDS lies in the unity of non-governmental organizations, families, governments and international donors. Non-governmental organizations need to collaborate and work with each other to prevent gaps and overlaps when educating and caring for people with HIV and AIDS. AIDS education in the community, in schools, in the industry and in churches, needs coordination. The left hand needs to know what the right hand is doing to prevent misinformation. Teamwork between clinicians, doctors, nurses, community workers, religious organizations, family and individuals with HIV and AIDS needs to happen. Universities must collaborate with each other in terms of research and education on HIV and AIDS. HIV is transmitted, not only sexually, but also through blood transfusions. Non-governmental organizations must work with the National Red Cross to make sure blood is safe. Other non-governmental organizations that do prevention on sexual transmission of AIDS need to involve other diseases such as tuberculosis, malaria, teen pregnancy prevention, etc. Other non-governmental organizations dealing with nutrition, clean water, sanitation and other factors that affect the immune system must collaborate with non-governmental organizations that deal with AIDS. National networks of non-governmental organizations also need to collaborate with other African countries and international bodies.

The third "C" is comprehensive strategy. HIV infection and AIDS cannot be addressed from only a clinical approach. A comprehensive strategy that will deal with the total person needs to be applied. You need to know where the person lives, what the person's housing is like, their nutrition, their water supply, their sanitation conditions, economic development, social structure, their family and community. When President Thabo Mbeki of South Africa, in his speech to the World AIDS Conference in Durban, emphasized poverty as an issue in dealing with HIV infection, unfortunately most people misunderstood his point of view. I disagree with him on other issues related to HIV and AIDS, but I agree with him that if Africa does not deal with the issue of poverty, every effort of prevention of HIV and care of persons will be a "band aid" and not a treatment of the core cause of broken immune systems. If people lose their homes when it rains because they live in cardboard houses, if people do not have clean water and better facilities for sanitation, if they do not have food, if they are unemployed and not educated, most of them tend to engage in risky behavior. This makes the infection of HIV and AIDS easier, especially when escort services take advantage of impoverished young girls and they turn to prostitution.

A comprehensive strategy is needed where non-governmental organizations dealing with AIDS organizations can be able to work with non-governmental organizations dealing with housing issues, hunger issues, family issues, church, government, and business. I think that a national coalition for HIV and AIDS has to have a comprehensive strategy. This coalition must include all of the sectors, including persons living with AIDS. More will be discussed in the next chapter where the role of the government is discussed.

When the non-governmental organizations that are involved in HIV and AIDS prevention, advocacy and care can avoid competition and complement each other, when they can avoid being manipulated by funding sources and can be motivated by the needs of the community, when they can become culturally sensitive, when they can collaborate with everyone involved with preventing HIV infection and care of persons with AIDS, and when they can plan a comprehensive strategy, we shall win the war against HIV infection and AIDS.

CHAPTER 6

The Role of the African Government

African governments differ from each other in terms of economy, infrastructure, population and their immediate needs. Most African countries are centralized and there is a long bureaucracy that paralyzes the delivery of systems. African governments own the hospitals and clinics, with the exception of a few missionary and private hospitals. Most African countries are going through what I call the "three Ts."

The first "T" is transition from old government to new government, and, in most cases, this process is difficult, depending on whether the transition was peaceful or was by military means. Also it depends on whether the former regime sabotaged the economy so that the incoming government starts with hardship. The critical questions during transition are: Is the new government capable to rule, to unite the country, and to move the country from conflict to peace? Is the government thriving on tribalism or nationalism? The transition is the most difficult time, as the masses want the government to deliver soon, and there is little capacity. On the other hand, the top governmental personnel are getting rich quickly with corruption here and there.

The second "T" is transformation, which is a difficult concept for some African governments. Is the government a servant of the people or the master of the people? During transformation, other governments are protecting the status quo and some are transforming the status quo. Transformation may have a few " labor pains" but it is worth the implementation. These transformations are needed in infrastructure, education, economy and culture. Transformation of the society will bring forth human rights, stability, and democracy.

The third "T" is transparency. Transparency is needed in African governments, so that people will be sympathetic to the government. It helps them understand its weaknesses and strengths. The government that is transparent consults with the civil society and is not ruled by a dictatorship. The government will not hide problems but acknowledge them and look for solutions. When the government is transparent it will win the trust of its citizens and it will be able to withstand external pressures.

The role of the government in Africa depends on whether it is socialist or capitalist or somewhere in the middle. In a socialist government, the government promises to provide everything–housing, health care, work, education, defense, and child-care–because the government owns the means of production. Is that practical? You be the judge. In capitalism, the government doesn't own everything; rather, ownership is encouraged. Business has the upper hand, which, if it is not well regulated, can exploit the workers. In social democratic countries, government tries to balance the socialist and the capitalist models. However, in countries like Angola, there have been conflicts of fighting either the system of capitalism or socialism. Generally, there are few countries that allow opposition parties on the table. Most countries arrest the opposition members and sabotage their efforts to organize, so that they flee into exile. Democracy without discipline and accountability is demonic and crazy (democrazy). The challenge facing governments in the fight of HIV and AIDS will be determined by the political and economical context and climate of the country. What is the priority? What comes first in the country? Is it a ceasefire, like in the Congo? Is it eliminating poverty or providing food, housing, education, jobs, clean water, a good sanitation? Is boosting the economy a priority? Can the governments with few resources make difficult choices between dealing with these many health problems, including malaria, TB, infant mortality due to diarrhea, and AIDS? Fortunately or unfortunately, depending on which side you are looking at it, HIV and AIDS has strong activists around the world, and they will make the Government listen and act.

Now the question is, should the African countries put HIV infection and AIDS on the back burner? Absolutely not. The government should join the individual, family, non-governmental organizations, churches, businesses, and international bodies in the fight against HIV. The approach will depend on the will of the political leaders and the resources they have, both financial and human. Unfortunately, there is the reality of demands from other illnesses that are curable, unlike AIDS. However, since most governments in Africa are centralized, they need to change priorities from building military machinery, and provide economic development, because there will be no army if everyone has died from AIDS. African countries need to continue with the philosophy of preventative measures because prevention is better than a cure, especially when resources are few.

Since there are more needs than resources, African governments need to step up more means of prevention. More resources should go towards prevention. Governments need to remove the stigma of AIDS, enacting laws that are not discriminatory. The government should have a task force look into HIV and AIDS prevention and care. Coordination of services between the Ministry of Health, medical professionals, public health institutions, ministry of welfare and social work, education, and NGOs, needs to be encouraged. Shouldn't indigenous doctors be included in the care system promoting alternative therapies? Governments need policies to encourage research. Government needs to provide resources for families with HIV and AIDS. It would cost less for orphans to be with their families rather than in an institution. More education and incentives are needed for promotion in the township and villages.

The mode of transmission of HIV is not only sexual but through blood transfusion. African governments have a responsibility for processing blood donations and banking blood products. It is not clear whether the blood used for transfusions in African countries is safe. Precautions need to be taken to make sure that people with high risk do not donate blood. Coordination of national societies with other Red Cross societies should be encouraged. According to the American Red Cross Research, in their international division in Washington, D.C., 28 African Red Cross societies are engaged in HIV prevention, care and support. These are Benin, Botswana, Burkina Faso, Cameroon, Central African Republic, Côte' d'Ivoire, Eritrea, Ethiopia, Ghana, Kenya, Lesotho, Malawi, Mali, Namibia, Niger, Nigeria, Rwanda, Senegal, Sierra Leone, Somalia, South Africa, Sudan, Swaziland Tanzania, Togo, Zambia and Zimbabwe. There are 5 African Red Cross Societies involved with gathering blood and testing for HIV. These are Benin, Botswana, Ethiopia, Sierra Leone, Swaziland and Togo. There are 15 countries involved with Blood Donor Recruitment, namely Botswana, Cape Verde, Ethiopia, Guinea, Guinea Bissau, Kenya, Lesotho, Malawi, Mozambique, Nigeria, Seychelles, Sierra Leone, Swaziland and Togo. Botswana is involved with voluntary counseling and testing.

What African governments are facing now is what happened to the

United States from 1984 to 1991. There was an urgency about AIDS education and care, but now, in the late nineties and 21st century, the urgency has dropped due to the development of antirectroviral drugs, which do not cure AIDS but stall the progression of the HIV infection. However, in some areas, infection is still rising. What should the government do? Government should make short and long term plans, have epidemiological studies to see which populations are at most risk, and provide resources. Some governments have policies that provide health care to citizens for free. While these policies are noble, the question is whether those governments can manage financially to give drugs free without breaking the country's economy. As Dr. Josef Decosas Director of Southern Africa in AIDS training programs wrote in the *New York Times* concerning antiretroviral drugs, "What good is a $300 antiretroviral package to the villager in Ghana with AIDS when Ghana's per capita income is $350 per year?" Also, how are the drugs going to be distributed?

African government needs the following programs for effective prevention, control and care of HIV and AIDS:
- Prevention programs that will include the education sector
- Prevention of mother to child transmission of HIV
- Safe blood transfusion
- Voluntary testing and counseling
- Screening and following up infected patients
- Access to medication
- Hospices for AIDS patients in later stages
- Support of families and orphans
- More funding

In the Abuja Conference in April, 2001, heads of African states pledged 15% of their budget to fund health services in their own countries.

Each country will need to assess its stability, resources and needs in order to form a comprehensive collaborating strategy for short-term and long-term goals. Support is needed from individuals, families, non-governmental organizations and international organizations. African governments need to work closely with the business community, especially pharmaceutical companies, concerning patent regulations on drugs. Also, governments need confidentiality policies that will protect those persons infected with HIV. Screening may be controversial, as it may raise ethical questions. How is screening done? Is there enough pre- and post- counseling done? When people test positive, do they have enough care for them? Should there be blind testing, especially for pregnant mothers? Does the government have mental health facilities for those people who may be suicidal after finding out that they're HIV positive? The African governments may need to decentralize their governance so that communities can be empowered to take care of themselves.

African governments need debt relief and cancellation so that they can use those funds to build infrastructure, provide education, and prevent disease, instead of increasing military spending and enriching themselves.

International support is expected to assist African governments in the economic policies and trade. The policies need to be fair. According to World Bank official aid to Sub-Sahara has fallen from US$32 per head in 1990 to US$19 by 1998 despite effective results in countries with sound economic policies. The Africa Growth and Opportunity Act has passed in the United States to boost African Trade. It needs to be implemented to assist the economy of African countries.

African countries also need to work through their regional political bodies, such as Southern African Development Community (SADC), Economic Council of West African States (ECOWAS), etc. to fight HIV and AIDS.

CHAPTER 7

The Role of the African Faith Communities

Africa has three major religious faiths: Christianity, African religions, and Islam. What is the role of these faith communities in regards to HIV and AIDS? The faith community has a divine mandate to give hope to the hopeless and help to helpless and healing to the sick. In the Christian faith community Jesus Christ is the center of the faith. His ministry consisted of preaching, teaching and healing. Matthew 16:18-19 states, "And I tell you that you are Peter and on this rock I will build my church and the gates of Hades will not overcome it. I will give you the keys of the kingdom of heaven, whatever you bind on earth will be bound in heaven." The church has the power. Here are the questions: Is the church aware of this power? Is the church using this power from God?

The power of God comes when people work in unity and not against one another. The issue is not that my denomination has a better true doctrine than yours. The critical issue is what is God saying to the church in Africa now when many people are dying of AIDS? Is there a word for salvation on the African continent? The answer is, yes, there is a word from God to the church, to be a power to overcome evil, to love unconditionally, and to prophesy when the people of God have gone astray. The church has the inspired scriptures according to I Timothy 3:16, "for profitable doctrine, for reproof, for correction, for instruction in righteousness, so that the people of God may be perfect, thoroughly furnished unto all good works."

When AIDS began in the '80s affecting homosexual men in America, the church was quick to judge that it was the wrath of God punishing them. Some churches were afraid to get involved. The church here is not a building but an assembly of God's people. I remember in 1986 when I was working with the Baltimore health department as a health educator specializing in AIDS education. It was not easy to convince the churches, especially Black churches, that HIV and AIDS was not a homosexual disease but a disease that can affect anyone who is exposed to HIV, either sexually, through intravenous drug use, blood transfusion or in childbirth, if the mother is HIV infected. During that time, pediatric AIDS was on the rise in the black community, as the heterosexual community was infected. Persons with HIV infection or with AIDS were afraid, angry, feeling guilty and were not dealing with anyone except those they trusted. They could not even tell their families and pastors if they were in church. Also, the pastors and ministers were not educated enough about the epidemic.

I was wearing two hats at the time—a minister and a public health educator. The question was, how do I reach my colleagues, especially pastors with AIDS education? I knew that if I could reach the pastors with the message, the congregation would follow. Fortunately, I was working with the health commissioner, the late Dr. Maxie Collier, who was not afraid to embrace the Health Ministry and bring it into the Health Department. As the first black health commissioner in the city, he had an understanding of the critical role the church can play, especially in the black community.

I was on the ministerial staff at the Bethel AME Church. The church had more than 5000 members at that time. My senior pastor was the Rev. John Bryant, now bishop in the AME church. I asked him if the church, since it was the largest in Baltimore, could sponsor a prayer breakfast for those infected with HIV or AIDS. He was concerned that it was a homosexual disease. We had a homosexual person who attended the church with female clothes. He had accepted Christ as a savior and changed. The church donated male clothing to him, and he eventually became a minister, Rev. G. But I had to do a one-on-one AIDS discussion with Rev. Bryant. I brought AIDS data to him, especially as it related to the black community, the drug using community and children. We had a substance-abuse ministry (Freedom Now) already, but the issue of sponsoring a citywide prayer breakfast was difficult at first. But, as he was a man who did not want to stand in the way when God calls someone to ministry in the Church, he agreed to co-sponsor the first citywide prayer breakfast in Baltimore. Since I had his name and the church as one of the sponsors, I approached other churches, starting with the churches that had substance-abuse ministries and other big churches. Many churches agreed to be co-sponsors. My friend and colleague, Rev. Mamie Williams, now Annapolis Superintendent of the United Methodist Church, was the chairperson of the Prayer Breakfast on AIDS.

When I thought my big hurdle was over because the Black churches were on my side, there was a challenge from the Baltimore City Health Department to choose the guest speaker for the prayer breakfast. One of my supervisors wanted a white homosexual man to be the guest speaker. I was not for the idea. Not that I was against the individual personally, but that it was not going to work, since the Black church was not embracing homosexual behavior and it would reinforce the idea that HIV is a homosexual disease. I was not willing to force the churches to accept homosexual behavior, since, to me, the issue was not about the homosexual lifestyle but about the prevention of the spread of HIV and AIDS through drug use in the heterosexual community, specifically the black community. That community was not being reached.

I proposed Mr. P, a young black man who was HIV-positive and a former drug user who was a very eloquent speaker. I had met him at an AIDS conference where he was the speaker. Finally we agreed to have him as the guest speaker. The prayer breakfast was successful. It had in attendance 150 pastors in Baltimore, for the first time embracing the HIV and AIDS epidemic. Our speaker, coming out of the black church, gave an excellent speech. His testimony was about his life. He took responsibility for his addiction, which made him become infected, and testified about his repentance, asking for forgiveness. He said it was now his ministry to educate young people about drug abuse and the spread of HIV and AIDS. In the prayer breakfast the Ministers saw one of their own. They could identify with him and see that it could have been their son or a member of their congregation infected with HIV or having AIDS.

We formed a coalition of churches working against AIDS and also my church created an AIDS ministry. What I learned from the churches' role with HIV and AIDS ministry is that the church has to be the church, and not compromise its moral authority when it stands for righteousness and compassion. In most cases, people mistake calling for righteousness and speaking against immorality and society as being judgmental, and having compassion for those who are infected through sexual behavior as condoning the sinful behavior. The AIDS educators must have a different curriculum for AIDS education in the Church. One script is not suitable for every aspect, especially when it comes to the question of how you prevent the spread of HIV. I had a tough time in the health department convincing my colleagues to include abstinence as another way of preventing HIV infection. The attitude was that abstinence is not realistic, since the majority of young people where having sex. I was encouraged by the few who where not, and I also believe that we can also motivate the ones who are having sex to be secondary virgins. I believe in young people, that if they are given another option, they may change their behavior.

One Baptist church in Baltimore had a seminar on AIDS. One of the nurses who was a member of that church invited the AIDS educator from one of the AIDS non-governmental organizations to give a presentation. The pastor, church deacons, missionaries and young people were present. The educator spoke about what AIDS is and the mode of transmission. When she talked about preventing the spread of HIV, she mentioned the use of condoms and masturbation. The pastor and the congregation were angry. They saw AIDS education as promoting promiscuity that is not allowed in the church. They were going to start an AIDS ministry, but they dropped it.

The nurse at the church was determined to start an AIDS ministry at that church, so she asked the pastor for a second chance to have seminar. Through prayer, the pastor agreed. This time the nurse invited me to speak. First, I knew I needed to talk to them in a language they could understand and to which they could relate. I used a Biblical story about the woman with the issue of blood for 12 years (Luke 8:43-44). AIDS is a blood-borne disease, hence we have to deal with it. I emphasized abstinence from sexual intercourse for the unmarried and a monogamous relationship for married people, as methods of prevention of HIV. I quoted I Corinthians 6:19, "Do you not know that your body is the temple of the Holy Spirit, who is in you, whom you have received from God?" I also spoke about walking in the purpose of God and that HIV should not interrupt that journey. They asked me questions and everyone was pleased. We began with a prayer and also ended with a prayer. That is very important when you are giving AIDS education in a church. If AIDS educators are afraid to pray, they can ask the members of the Church to do it.

When teaching about HIV infection, it is also important to know your audience. People who have just found out that they are HIV-positive go through different emotions: denial, anger, blaming themselves and others, fear, bitterness, isolation, suicidal ideation and rejection by their loved ones, especially if they were drug users or homosexual. When people are infected with HIV or having AIDS, they are hurting. They are like a man wounded in the Good Samaritan story in the Bible (Luke 10:25-37). The church should embrace the people with HIV with compassion and love.

I've had many experiences where I was called to the hospital to pray or give words of encouragement. One of them was when I was called to the University of Maryland Hospital in Baltimore to visit a person who belonged to Bethel AME church where I was one of ministerial staff. During my lunchtime from the Health Department, I went to the nurse's station. He was screaming and cursing in his room. I knocked and with a loud voice he said, "Who is that?" I told him my name and that I was from Bethel AME Church. He said to me, "Come in."

I went in and he was lying on the bed. I greeted him and he responded. I asked him if there was something he would like to have. "Nothing," he replied. He requested a prayer and I prayed. After prayer, he was calm. He started to talk. I was listening attentively. In our conversation I sensed trauma, pain, isolation, guilt, and fear, especially of death. I asked him if it was all right to read Scripture to him. He said it was fine. I read him Psalm 23, "The Lord is my shepherd I shall not want . . ." I held his hand and shared with him that God loved him and we also loved him. My time was over and I said goodbye. He asked me if I was coming the following day. I said, "Yes." I could see a smile on his face. He was happy that I promised to come. I went back to work.

That was Monday. I began reflecting on the visit. When I went into the room, he was screaming and cursing and when I left after prayer and reading the scripture he had a smile on his face. That was the manifestation of God's power when we can allow God to use us.

Tuesday, again during lunchtime, I went to the hospital to see him. On my arrival, I found he was with his lover. He introduced me to him. They were holding hands. I asked if I had come at an inappropriate time and if they needed privacy. They said, no, and his lover said he was on his way out. He stood up and said goodbye.

I asked him how he was feeling and he said he was feeling weak. I asked if he was ready for prayer. He said he was. I held his hand and we prayed and read Scripture, Psalm 121, "I will lift up mine eyes to the hills, where does my help comes from?" We talked about the power of God to forgive and bless. He said he had done many wrong things in his life, and he was not sure whether they could be forgiven. I told him that every one of us has wronged God. I shared with him Romans 3:23, "For all have sinned and come short of the glory of God." I also read him the Scripture Isaiah 1 verse 18, "and though your sins are like scarlet and they shall be as white as snow." I told him that everyone of us has sinned and we come to God to ask for forgiveness so that we can move into a new life with God. I shared with him that God through His love did his share. He gave us His son, Jesus Christ to save us, but it is up to us to accept the love and the gift of God. It is not about what I did yesterday, but it is about what I can do today to change my future. I asked him to think about it and my time was up. As I was leaving, he asked again if I was coming the following day, Wednesday, and I said yes.

I left, and on my way to the elevator, the nurse came to me and said, "Rev., since you've come to visit Mr. S, he has changed. He is no longer screaming, rude, and blaming everyone. My response was, "Praise the Lord, continue to pray for him." I departed. On my way back to work at the Health Department, it was again confirmed in my heart that health is not only physical and mental but also spiritual, and I began to hope we could start tapping the spiritual issues in our health education. In my prayer and meditation I started to pray for those in a similar situation similar to Mr. S who may not have a minister to take the time to heal their souls and encourage their spiritual journey.

The following day, Wednesday, I went again to the hospital. This time Mr. S was highly spirited and doing much better. "Rev.," he said, "I'm grateful to you that you can take time every day to see me. I feel better. It's such a relief to know that some people care." I said, "Thank you. Remember that it is God who first loved and cared for us. We're just instruments of this provision of love and care." We prayed, and he showed me a smile and kept on saying many times that he was feeling better. I read him the Scripture, Psalm 91, verses 9-16, "For God will command his angels concerning you to guard you in all your ways and they will lift you up in their hands so that you will not strike your foot against a stone." I held his hands and we prayed and then I said goodbye. I was not afraid to hold his hands when we prayed because I knew you cannot get HIV by touching. He was happy and he smiled and said, "Rev., Will I see you tomorrow? As usual I said, "Yes, we will meet tomorrow."

Thursday came, and during lunchtime I went to the hospital. I went to the room and he was not there. Immediately I thought maybe he was discharged or transferred somewhere. I went to the nurses' station and asked where he was. The nurse told me that he had passed away that day and left a message with his sister to let me know that he was at peace with God. My heart was filled joy. I thank God for being a part of his love manifestation and for the opportunity God gave me with Mr. S. I will treasure it.

The ministry encouraged me to also grow spiritually. I was able to realize that there is more in the human spirit than the labels we put on people or that they put on themselves. I also learned that we must minister according to the needs of the individual and not according to our needs. I share this experience, not to boast, but to inspire God's servants in Africa that God can use us according to His calling.

When dealing with HIV infection and AIDS we cannot conform to the world, but we have to transform the world (Romans 12:2). I am aware that the church in Africa is divided into denominations and also into political wings, the right wing and the left wing. Unfortunately, HIV does not care much about which denomination or political wing it attacks. We, as the church, should embrace all denominations and both wings to cover every territory. I had lunch with two South African ministers. I asked the one who was very active during Apartheid and even after to share some thoughts about the role of the church in the prevention of HIV and care for people with AIDS. He said he does not want to do anything with AIDS, and many ministers feel that way. I asked him what was the reason for feeling this way. He told me the experience he had.

There was a rally in the township on AIDS education. They asked him to come and open the ceremony in prayer. He went there and prayed and the Kwato musical group came and sang. They started opening boxes of condoms and throwing them to the people who attended the rally. He saw young people catching them and some thought that they were balloons and started putting them in their mouth and blowing air into them. He said he was disgusted about the whole AIDS education issue and decided that he was not going to continue participating in those rallies and AIDS education. I understood what he meant and I discussed with him that not to participate was still not right, as he would be faced with burying others who may not have had an opportunity to be loved and cared for by God's messengers. He understood that we, as the church, need to get involved with the AIDS epidemic.

We found that there is a need to educate the church and for the government and the non-governmental organizations to be sensitive to the biblical mandate of the Church to promote purity and chastity (Matthew 15:16-20), "but things that come out of the mouth, come from the heart and these make a man unclean." For out of the heart come evil thoughts: murder, adultery, sexual immorality, theft, false testimony and slander. Also the church has a biblical mandate to be compassionate (Luke 10:25-37). The story of the Good Samaritan who saw the wounded man on the road where Church people passed by and did not help, a priest and a Levite, but a Good Samaritan took care of him. Those who are wounded by the infection of HIV and AIDS need compassion. We should not impose our faith, but minister as those who have the disease allow. God will open the door and He will guide us if we listen and do not rush Him.

Africa has also Islam as a religion of the people. My observation is that HIV infection and AIDS is reported in Sub-Saharan African countries. African countries north of the Sub-Sahara, which are Islamic, have not reported HIV infection and AIDS as much (see pp. 63-63). This might be because Islamic religion restricts female and male relationships outside of marriage and they promote marriage at the young age and most of those marriages are arranged. More studies are needed to research those communities.

Collaboration between the Christian, Islamic, and African religions is needed to agree on some spiritual mandate, whether it be from the Bible, Quaran, or African Spiritism. The African religion includes God who is referred to in different names in different languages. In South Africa God is known as Modimo, Thixo, Unkulunkulu, in Zimbabwe Mudzimo, in Tanzania Mungu, in Nigeria Chineke, Oluwa. The African religions make use of possessions, experiences, rituals, and ancestral spirits, who are the spirits of people who died physically but live in spirit and continue a personal relationship with those who are living.

In 1978, I was detained for anti-apartheid activities in South Africa. I was put in solitary confinement for 21 days in the jail. Of course I prayed to God through Christ, as I was a Christian. I did not know that my maternal grandmother's sister, my mother's aunt in the village, planted a small plant the day she received the news that I had been arrested. Every morning and every night she went to the plant and talked to my deceased grandparents and great grandparents to intervene for me. She could never understand why a person who hadn't killed someone or stolen could be arrested. She did not understand the internal security laws in South Africa. What she was concerned about was that she needed to pray and talk to her family who had passed away so that I could be released.

Indeed, I was released. I lived in Soweto. I was asked by my family to go and visit all the relatives in the rural areas in Northern Transvaal, now Northern Province, so that they could see I had been released. I visited my great aunt who was about 70 years and the only Matriarch left. When she heard that I was released, she cried and held me and took me to the outside to where she planted the little tree. She held me with her hand and thanked the ancestors for my release. She told me that she planted it as a reminder to her that I was in jail. Now that I was released, she plucked it out. I hugged her and I felt the power of love. I learned that she knew how to communicate with Modimo or God.

There are many people in Africa who still believe in ancestors. The question is, how can we work together to prevent HIV and AIDS? Instead of merely condomizing Africa, I believe there are other spiritual, African ways in which we can come together to bring hope, help and healing to Africa. I am encouraged by the Scripture in II Chronicles 7:14, "If my people in Africa, who are called by my name shall humble themselves and pray and seek my face and turn from their wicked ways, then I will hear from heaven and will forgive their sins and will heal their land." God will indeed heal Africa of its ills.

CHAPTER 8

The Role of the International Community

In March, 1991, I was employed as the National Coordinator of the National Coordinating Council for Repatriation of South African Exiles. In that role, I learned how the International community can rally under one cause–repatriation of exiles from all over the world back to South Africa. I worked closely with the United Nations High Commission for Refugees, another division of the United Nations. I worked with foreign governments through their embassies in South Africa, the European Union, The World Council of Churches, denominational churches through their missions, and numerous international non-governmental organizations from different countries. They assisted by supplying monetary and human resources.

I believe the same model can be used where international agencies, foreign governments, international non-governmental organizations, and the religious community can assist in the prevention of HIV infection and care of persons with AIDS. In April, 2001, The United Nations, through the leadership of General Secretary Kofi Annan, facilitated a conference with the African Heads of State in Abuja, Nigeria, to involve them in the AIDS epidemic.

The World Health Organization has several projects in Africa to fight AIDS. Foreign aid from foreign governments depends on the policies of that government. The question is whether aid is really aid to help and empower the people or does it merely create dependency? Can the projects be sustainable after the aid is gone?

International aid always has a political "string" attached. Some foreign governments may not give aid if it is not in the interest of its government. However some will give on a humanitarian basis. International aid would be better implemented if African nationals are involved, as they know the language and the culture of the people. Aid should not be dictated to African countries but given in a collaboration that considers the priorities of the countries to whom the aid is being given.

The financial international organizations, like the World Bank and the International Monetary Fund, have sent aid to Africa at high cost and interest. Presently most African countries are unable to pay back the loans. Not all is the fault of these international financial organizations, some African leaders have misused those funds, enriching themselves and their families. There was Jubilee 2000 Movement to petition the foreign governments and those institutions to cancel the African debt so that those countries could be able to finance developments and prevent diseases, such as AIDS, Malaria and TB. The debt relief and cancellation is continuing its activism and there is collaboration with other organizations involved with HIV and AIDS, hunger and the environment.

In the fight of HIV and AIDS, the Western governments need to revisit cancellation and relief of debt while ensuring that money is not spent on the military and corruption.

The international pharmaceutical companies have exploited Africa, charging excessive amounts for drugs and refusing the development of generic drugs in the name of protecting their patents. The AIDS activists put much pressure on the pharmaceutical companies, and they dropped the legal charges against the government of South Africa. The pharmaceutical companies have now repented and say that their companies were not geared for developing countries. They have pledged to give drugs for free and they are collaborating with the Makerere University in Uganda to train doctors to administer those drugs. Also, recently, the president of South Africa, Thabo Mbeki, while attending the UN Conference on Global AIDS in June, 2001, met with the pharmaceutical companies in the U.S. to work with them in capacity building and the cost of drugs.

The multinational companies need to be involved in the fight of HIV and AIDS. Their workers are affected by the epidemic. Health insurance for workers is necessary. HIV and AIDS policies at the workplace are necessary. AIDS education is imperative to avoid discrimination of workers by other workers or managers. When I was working with The Health Department in 1986, there was a policy to educate every employee about HIV and AIDS. I went to every division of the Health Department to do AIDS education. Every employee signed an attendance sheet. It took me four months. The lecture was two hours. We were able to deal with fears about how you can get or not get HIV. Early AIDS education and testing of employees can help the company in the long run. Employees who test positive should not be fired, as this will make HIV testing difficult. Abstinence and condom use are options to prevent HIV, and workers should be encouraged to take these precautions. Every company will formulate its policies according to their work conditions.

The United States has passed the Africa Growth Opportunity Act (AGOA). While some people have criticized the Act, the African Diplomats have hailed the Act as the beginning of equal partnership in trade with the U.S. They say that the Act will benefit trade in Africa and boost the economy to eradicate poverty. We hope that those involved with international trade will not exploit the workers, but give them decent living wages and health care. Also, that these companies will be environmentally friendly by not polluting the air and water. The United States has pledged $200 million for HIV assistance in Africa.

The European Union (EU) has decided to give assistance to Africa. On November, 2000, the Council of Development Ministers adopted a resolution on combating the transmissible disease. The Nice European Council adopted a comprehensive approach on optimization of help and development policies, reduction of cost of drugs, and research and medicines, and social dimensions of infectious diseases. The European Union also endorsed The Institution of Global HIV/AIDS and the Health Fund. The European governments also pledged individually to assist the African countries in the AIDS epidemic. They will assist non-governmental organizations, community based organizations, HIV voluntary and confidential counseling and testing, HIV prevention of mother-to-child transmission, HIV/AIDS information, education and communication, people living with AIDS, sexually transmitted diseases, tuberculosis, antiretroviral therapy, commercial sex workers, and implementing agencies.

International philanthropic foundations also have pledged to assist the African NGOs to prevent HIV infection and to care for persons living with AIDS and orphans.

The United Nations convened the 26th Special Session of the General Assembly on June 25-27, 2001, at the headquarters in New York to mobilize the UN member states to address the problem of HIV/AIDS in the world, particularly in Africa. A UN declaration was agreed upon the implementation of policies as well as the development of the Health Fund. The UN General Secretary, Kofi Annan, promised to work also with the business community to build the Health Fund. UN member states pledged money to the fund. The gifts will be tax deductible. The declaration also noted that, at the end of the year 2000, 36.1 million people, worldwide, were living with AIDS, 90% in the developing countries and 75% in Sub-Sahara Africa.

CHAPTER 9

The Prophetic Sermon on Mt. Kilimanjaro

TEXT: Ezekiel 37:1-13 and Matthew 5:1-12

Ezekiel 37:

V.3. He asked me, "Son of man, can these bones live?" I said, "O Sovereign Lord, you alone know."

V.4. Then he said to me, "Prophesy to these bones and say to them, "Dry bones, hear the word of the Lord.

V.5. This is what the Sovereign Lord said to these bones, "I will make breath enter you and you will come to life.

V.6. "I will attach tendons to you and make flesh come upon you and cover you with skin. I will put breath in you, and you will come to life. Then you will know that I am the Lord."

V.14. "I will put my Spirit in you and you will live, and I will settle you in your own land. Then you will know that I the Lord have spoken, and I have done it," declares the Lord.

Matthew 5:

V.1. Now when He (Jesus) saw the crowds, He went up on the mountainside and sat down. His disciples came to him

V.2. and he began to teach them, saying

V.3. Blessed are the poor in spirit, for theirs is the kingdom of heaven.

I have just completed the Bible study on the books of the prophets at the Lord's church, Kalafong AME, where I am a servant. The book of the prophet Ezekiel struck me, especially Chapter 37. I could identify with him when he was in the valley and saw many dry bones. When I look at Africa, seeing young and old people infected and dying of AIDS, young children becoming orphans and infected: that is dry bones. Some governments do not know what to do, some are engaged in wars, some are overwhelmed economically still facing to pay international debt: that is dry bones. Young children are made child soldiers, engaged in wars they do not understand, children are amputated and young girls are turning to be prostitutes: that is dry bones. Virgins are raped because of misinformation about cure of AIDS: that is dry bones.

Immorality, promiscuity: that is dry bones. Poor housing, poor sanitation, poor water supply, (now in some parts of Africa water is privatized): that is dry bones. Poverty, unemployment, greed and corruption: that is dry bones. Exploitation of natural resources, low GNP's: that is dry bones.

The question is, can these dry bones in Africa live again? Can Africa, the cradle of civilization in ancient times live again? We read of Timbaktu, the first University in Africa. We read of Imhotep the father of medicine. Can Africa with its potential of people and natural resources live again?

In verse 11, I can hear people in Africa saying, "Our bones are dried up, our hope is gone and we are cut off with the HIV and AIDS epidemic."

I am encouraged, and I know that Africa can live again. There are three points to understand for Africa to live again.

1. **Hope.** Hope is a feeling that what is wanted will happen. We want Africa to live again and it will happen. In verse 12, The Sovereign Lord says, "My people, I am going to open your graves and bring you back to the land. Verse 14,"I will put my Spirit in you and you will live." These words give us hope that Africa will live again. Reverend Jessie Jackson always says, "Keep hope alive." Edward Mute wrote the words of the great hymn of the Church. "My hope is built on nothingness than on Jesus' blood and righteousness . . . On Christ the solid rock I stand, all other is sinking sand." In South Africa, we have a Sesotho gospel song "Ke tshepile wena. Ha ra ditsietsi, ha ra mahlomoleng ke tshepile wena Jesu." The meaning of the song is, "My hope is in you. In my troubles, trial and tribulation, my hope is in Jesus." Hope is going to give us faith. With faith we shall not despair. With faith we shall move the mountain (I Corinthians 13:2). With faith we shall know that "One who is in us is greater than the one in the world" (I John 4:4).

2. **Help.** We not only need hope but we need help and action. The psalmist says, "In my distress, I talked to the Lord. I cried for help (Psalm 18:6). My help comes from the Lord, the Maker of heaven and earth (Psalm 121:2). God is our refuge and strength, an ever present help in trouble, therefore we will not fear, though the earth give away and the mountains fall into the heart of the sea, though its waters roar

and foam and the mountains quake with surging (Psalm 46:1-3), though people are dying of AIDS and we are left with orphans, though still people are not taking precautions to protect themselves sexually because of lack of information or disbelief of the information, though there is lack of access to drugs for those who need it, especially those infected mothers. Though it seems discouraging and depressing, there is a river whose streams make glad the city of God, the place where the Most High dwells (Psalm 46:4). God will help us to help others. We can help by giving our time, our talent and our treasures to prevent the spread of HIV and AIDS. God has already raised people to help as educators, caregivers clinicians, researchers, prophets, priests, politicians, business leaders, activists, families and friends to help. These people help because they are filled with Hope.

3. Healing. Hope in God, help from God leads to healing our souls. When our souls are healed, our minds and bodies will be healed. According to Strong's *Exhaustive Concordance*, there are 156 scriptures about heal, healing, healed, healer and health. Jesus' ministry was about preaching, teaching and healing. In some cases, persons infected by HIV and have AIDS are not killed by the virus but by psycho-social-spiritual factors. They are in trauma, angry, bitter, guilt, fear, rejected by family, depressed and thinking of committing suicide. These feelings affect their immune systems. There is a message of hope that will bring healing of the spirit first. "The Lord will forgive all our sins and heal all our diseases (Psalm 103:3).

The gospels are filled with the ministry of Jesus' healing. Mark records extensively these ministries. The healing of a man with leprosy, Peter's mother-in-law, the Centurion's servant, the paralytic, the man with the evil spirit, the women who had bleeding for 12 years, the Syrophoenician woman possessed by demons, the deaf and the mute man, the blind man and the boy possessed by demons (Mark 1:21 - 9:30). All the time, Jesus cured many who had diseases, sicknesses and evil spirits. The blind received sight, the lame walked, those who had leprosy were cured, the deaf heard, the dead were raised and the good news was preached (Luke 7:21-23).

Jesus is the same yesterday, today and forever (Hebrew 13:8). God still works the same as He worked during Ezekiel's and Jesus' time. God has already breathed His Spirit on the dry bones in Africa and they shall live again.

We shall live again because Jesus is on the Kilimanjaro Mountain saying:

Blessed are the poor in spirit, with guilt, fear, anger, depression, suicidal ideation, rejected and neglected by family and governments because they are infected with HIV and have AIDS, for theirs is the kingdom of God.

Blessed are those who mourn their sons and daughters, their husbands and wives, their aunts and uncles, their grandchildren, their lovers, their friends, their country men and women who have died of AIDS, for they shall be comforted.

Blessed are the meek, those who have compassion, those who are not judgmental, those who have dedicated themselves to educate and minister to those suffering from AIDS, for they will inherit the earth.

Blessed are those who hunger after righteousness, who are responsible with their sexual behaviors, who are monogamous in their marriage, those who are not abusive in their relationship, those who respect women and children, those who govern with ethics, for they shall be filled.

Blessed are the merciful, those who are willing to forgive their children who were engaged in high risk behaviors, international government who are willing to relieve and cancel the debt of the African governments, those pharmaceutical companies who will choose passion over profits for access of drugs, for they shall be shown mercy.

Blessed are the pure in heart, those who have invited God to rule their hearts, those who have decided not to have sex until marriage, those who stand on righteousness and justice, those who do not discriminate because of the disease, for they shall see God.

Blessed are the peacemakers, those governments that promote human rights, that understand that they can solve political problems without violence, those governments that reduce their military budgets and increase economic and social development, those governments that do not exchange diamonds for military weapons, those who do not buy diamonds to fuel war in Africa, for they will be called the sons and daughters of the living God.

Blessed are those who are persecuted for not being politically correct but prophetically correct, who stand against immorality, promiscuity, pornography and corruption in government, for theirs is the kingdom of heaven.

Blessed are you, you, you, when you have hope in the Spirit of God and are willing to help in the healing of persons living with HIV and AIDS. These bones in Africa shall live again. With God's power we shall conquer HIV and AIDS. AMEN. AMEN. AMEN.

CHAPTER 10

A Prayer for Africa

If my people, who are called by my name will humble themselves and pray and seek my face and turn from their wicked ways, then will I hear from heaven and will forgive their sin and will heal their land" (II Chronicles 7:14) KJV.

In Southern Africa, they call you Modimo (Sesotho, Setswana, Sepedi), Unkulunkulu (isiZulu), Thixo (isiXhosa), in East Africa, they call you Mungu (Swahili), in West Africa Oluwa (Yoruba), Chineke (Ibo). In North Africa, they call you Allah. We all agree that you are our creator, out of nothing, from dust you made us in your image. We know and believe that you are omniscient, you know everything and all things. You are omnipotent, you have all power over your creation. You are omnipresent, you are everywhere, every place at once, watching over us and feeling our sufferings. We know you as the bread of life, for when we were hungry, you fed us. We know you as the Living Water, for when we were thirsty, you quenched our thirst. We know you as the great Counselor, because you regulated our minds when we were confused. Yes, we know you as our advocate because when we were in trouble, you gave us an acquittal. Yes, you are a great physician, for you have healed others and you still continue to heal.

Prophet Isaiah in the 53rd chapter and the 5th verse says by your son's wounds, we are healed. We come with holy boldness before your throne, we come with intercessory prayer, for our brothers and sisters, especially those living with AIDS and those infected with HIV in the Motherland Africa.

We are praying for our brothers and sisters who are gasping for their last breaths because of the disease, AIDS. Save their souls like one of the thieves on the cross, remember them in your paradise.

We are praying for our brothers and sisters who are on the battlefield with this disease. Instill hope, love and compassion for them.

We are praying for our brothers and sisters whose loved ones have died or are suffering from this disease, AIDS. Comfort them with your Holy Spirit.

We are praying for our brothers and sisters who are infected with HIV but do not have the symptoms of AIDS. Extinguish the fire of guilt, anger, fear, hopelessness, despair and instill forgiveness, joy, peace and faith in their hearts.

We pray for those who are not yet infected to be sexually responsible. Give them the power and strength to change and overcome sexual behaviors that put them at risk of the disease.

We pray for community health educators to impart the knowledge, facts about HIV and AIDS simple and clearly.

We pray for the clinicians, nurses, doctors who are risking their lives every day to care for persons with AIDS, to be sensitive and compassionate.

We pray for scientists who are working on the development of a vaccine and other drugs to cure AIDS. Give them the breakthrough to cure this disease.

We pray for the indigenous African doctors, to whom, before the western medicine, you gave wisdom to know the herbs that healed people. Work with them to discover other herb therapies to prevent and cure this disease.

We pray for the pharmaceutical companies to move away from greed and embrace compassion. Help them, O God, to have the resources to find new drug inventions but not at the expense of social responsibility within the industry.

We pray for the government leaders in Africa, give them the wisdom of Solomon so that they can know and understand how to provide for the needs of the people and create a balance in provision of resources between the military and education, healthcare and employment.

We pray for the church, the mosque, synagogues, especially the leaders, to be compassionate, caring, to preach, teach and heal the people of God. Help the church to balance the prophetic and the compassionate Word of God.

We pray for Your Spirit to help us know how to warn people about the consequences of the immoral life styles and also embrace compassion for those who have the disease.

We pray for the African family, to keep positive culture and values of respect for each other, not hurting each other, whether it is one's wife, husband, son, daughter, sister or brother, nephew, niece or cousin. Stop the demonic spirit of rape prevailing in community in Your Holy name. The African family, because of the concept of extended family, has shown sensitivity in caring for one another, widows and orphans. Help us, O God, to forsake the culture that is detrimental and destructive to the African family and help us to keep the parts of the culture that made us royal people of the Timbaktu.

We pray for the international community to assist us in the fight of the disease. We pray that they shall not be patriarchal, patronizing, be culturally sensitive with their aid.

We pray for the youth of Africa, future leaders of the continent that they may not be trapped in sexual desires that will squash their future dreams.

We pray, O God, because we believe in your word which says, "If my people who are called by my name shall humble themselves, pray and seek my face, [and seek my presence in their souls, in their minds and their social setting,] and turn away from their wickedness, I shall hear from heaven and heal their land" (I Chronicles 7:14).

Help us, O God, to move away from our wicked ways of unbelief, hatred to those who are suffering from the disease, judgmental spirit for those who are suffering from the disease, wicked ways in insensitivity, wicked ways of exploiting the young illiterate girls by making them products to sell their bodies for little money instead of providing education to liberate them from poverty, wicked ways of sexual behaviors that are detrimental to the fabric of our society.

Hear our prayers, heal our souls, heal our minds, Heal, O God, our bodies, Heal, O God, our families, Heal, O God, our governments, Heal, O God, our drug companies, Heal our health care providers, Heal, O God, our religious institutions, Heal, O God, the international bodies in their assistance. Heal us, Heal us, Heal us we pray.

Your African son, Enoch Sontonga composed an African prayer that is sung in Africa in isiXhoso and sesotho

Nkosi sikeleli' Afrika...	Lord bless Africa...
Maliphakamiswe upondo lwayo	May her horn be raised.
Izwa imithandzo yethu.	Hear our prayers.
Nkosi Sikeleli' I Afrika.	Lord bless Africa.
Woza uMoya uingcwele.	Come Holy Spirit.
Morena boloka setshaba sa heso.	God protect our nation.
O fedise dintwa le matswenyeho.	Stop the wars and sufferings.
O seboloke. Setshab asa heso.	Protect our nation.
Ma kube njalo. Ma kube njalo.	Let it be, Let it be.
Kude kube nguna phakade.	Forever and ever.

AMEN, AMEN AND AMEN.

APPENDIX A:

Excerpt From HIV/AIDS Population Impact Chart, Department Of Economic And Social Affairs, Population Division, 2001

	Total population (thousands) 2001	Adults (15-49 years) living with HIV/AIDS 1999 Number (thousands)	Adults (15-49 years) living with HIV/AIDS 1999 Percentage	AIDS deaths (thousands) 1999	AIDS orphans (thousands) 1999	Life expectancy at birth (years) 2000-2005 with AIDS	Life expectancy at birth (years) 2000-2005 without AIDS[1]	Government level of concern about AIDS	Blood screening	Screening high-risk groups	Information/ education campaign	Promoting condom use
	(1)	(2)	(3)	(4)	(5)	(6)	(7)	(8)	(9)	(10)	(11)	(12)
AFRICA												
Eastern Africa												
Burundi	6 502	340	11.3	39	150	41	52	Major	..	..	..	..
Comoros	727	<1	0.1	..	..	61	-	..	..	..	..	..
Djibouti	644	35	11.8	3	6	41	52	Minor	..	Yes	Yes	Yes
Eritrea	3 816	49	2.9	..	..	52	56	..	..	..	..	..
Ethiopia	64 459	2 900	10.6	280	903	43	53	Major	Yes	Yes	Yes	Yes
Kenya	31 293	2 000	14.0	180	547	49	66	Major	Yes	Yes	Yes	Yes
Madagascar	16 437	10	0.2	<1	2	54	-	..	..	..	..	..
Malawi	11 572	760	16.0	70	276	39	53	Major	Yes	Yes	Yes	Yes
Mauritius	1 171	<1	0.1	..	..	72	-	Major	..	..	..	..
Mozambique	18 644	1 100	13.2	98	248	38	49	..	..	..	..	..
Rwanda	7 949	370	11.2	40	172	41	51	Major	..	..	..	..
Seychelles	81	..	..	..	..	..	..	..	..	..	..	..
Somalia	9 157	..	..	..	..	49	54	..	..	..	..	..
Uganda	24 023	770	8.3	110	997	46	59	Major	Yes	Yes	Yes	Yes
United Rep. of Tanzania	35 965	1 200	8.1	140	667	51	59	Major	Yes	Yes	Yes	Yes
Zambia	10 649	830	20.0	99	447	42	60	Major	Yes	Yes	Yes	Yes
Zimbabwe	12 852	1 400	25.1	160	624	43	69	..	..	..	..	..
Middle Africa												
Angola	13 527	150	2.8	15	63	46	48	..	..	..	..	..
Cameroon	15 203	520	7.7	52	181	50	59	..	Yes	..	..	..
Central African Republic	3 782	230	13.8	23	70	44	55	Major	..	..	Yes	Yes
Chad	8 135	88	2.7	10	42	46	49	..	..	..	..	..
Congo	3 110	82	6.4	9	35	52	59	..	..	..	..	..
D. Rep. of the Congo	52 522	100	5.1	95	464	52	58	Major	..	..	..	..
Equatorial Guinea	470	1	0.5	<1	<1	52	-	..	..	..	..	..
Gabon	1 262	22	4.2	2	6	53	58	Major	..	..	..	..
Sao Tome and Principe	140	..	..	..	..	..	..	Major	..	..	..	..

Northern Africa											
Algeria	30 841	11	0.1	:	:	70	-	Minor	Yes	Yes	Yes
Egypt	69 080	8	0.0	:	:	68	-	:	:	:	:
Libyan Arab Jamahiriya	5 408	1	0.1	:	:	71	-	:	:	:	:
Morocco	30 430	5	0.0	:	:	69	-	Major	Yes	Yes	Yes
Sudan	31 809	140	1.0	:	:	57	-	:	:	:	:
Tunisia	9 562	2	0.0	:	:	71	-	:	:	:	:
Southern Africa											
Botswana	1 554	280	35.8	24	55	36	70	Major	Yes	Yes	Yes
Lesotho	2 057	240	23.6	16	29	40	64	Major	:	:	:
Namibia	1 788	150	19.5	18	53	44	64	Major	Yes	Yes	Yes
South Africa	43 792	4 100	19.9	250	371	47	66	:	:	:	:
Swaziland	938	120	25.3	7	11	38	63	Major	:	:	:
Western Africa											
Benin	6 446	67	2.5	6	17	54	57	Minor	:	:	:
Burkina Faso	11 856	330	6.4	43	212	48	56	Major	Yes	Yes	Yes
Cape Verde	437	:	:	:	:	71	-	:	:	:	:
Côte d'Ivoire	16 349	730	10.8	72	287	48	59	:	:	:	:
Gambia	1 337	12	2.0	1	6	47	49	:	:	:	Yes
Ghana	19 734	330	3.6	33	119	57	62	Major	Yes	Yes	Yes
Guinea	8 274	52	1.5	6	21	49	-	Major	Yes	No	Yes
Guinea-Bissau	1 227	13	2.5	1	4	45	48	:	:	:	:
Liberia	3 108	37	2.8	5	20	56	59	:	:	:	:
Mali	11 677	97	2.0	10	32	52	55	:	:	:	:
Mauritania	2 747	6	0.5	<1	2	52	-	:	:	:	:
Niger	11 227	61	1.4	7	22	46	-	Major	Yes	Yes	Yes
Nigeria	116 929	2 600	5.1	250	971	52	58	:	:	:	:
Senegal	9 662	76	1.8	8	29	54	-	:	:	:	:
Sierra Leone	4 587	65	3.0	8	36	41	43	:	:	:	:
Togo	4 657	120	6.0	14	63	52	59	:	:	:	:

NOTES

1. Nkosi Johnson is the young boy who championed the cause of AIDS in South Africa. Naming a child is important in Africa. In most cases your name resembles your personality. Nkosi is a word in isiZulu and isiXhosa, which means "king" "Lord". Nkosi Johnson was really a king in the world for what he stood for.
2. Mount Kilimanjaro is the highest mountain in Africa. It is in the North East of Tanzania. It is 19,340ft (5895m). New Webster College Dictionary.
3. Population estimates for mid-1999. World Bank Statistical Information Management and Analysis data base (SIMA) also UN Population and Vital Statistics.
4. GNP per capita figures in US dollars are calculated according to World Bank Atlas.
5. Primary school enrollment in Africa. Data from United Nations, Education, Scientific and Cultural Organization. (UNESCO)
6. African countries and regions. United Nations, Division of Population and Department of Economic and Social Affairs. 2001.
7. Languages in Africa. African Heritage Education and Research Institute. Baltimore.
8. United Nations, Division of AIDS. UNAIDS, AIDS Epidemic Update December 2000.
9. Scriptures are quoted from the Holy Bible in King James Version and New International Version.
10. Virus and AIDS. Fan H.; R.F. Conner, and L. P. Villarreal, (2000) *The Biology of AIDS*. Sudbury MA: Jones and Bartlett.
11. William B. and S. Knight (1994) *Healing for Life: Wellness and the Art of Living*. Pacific Grove, CA: Brooks Cole Publishing Company.
12. Edlin G., Golanty E., and K.M. Brown (1997) *Essentials for Health and Wellness* Sudsbury, MA: Jones and Bartlett Publishers.
13. Safety of Blood. American Red Cross, International HIV Division Washington, DC.
14. It takes a Village. *New York Times:* http://www.nytimes.com. Searchable Website for New York Times.
15. South African President Thabo Mbeki' Press Conference at the National Press Club live on C-Span, June 27, 2001.

16. The Special Session of General Assembly of the United Nations in June 2001.
17. French policy on International Co-operation in the fight against HIV/AIDS in the developing countries.
18. Water Privatization in Ghana. National Forum on Water Privatization, Accra Ghana: May 16 through 19.
http://www.challengeglobalization.org and public services.
19. The prayer song that became the African National Anthem. Nkosi sikeleli'Africa. (God bless Africa.)
20. A horn is a powerful symbol of power in Africa.

ABOUT THE AUTHOR

Rev. Dr. Mankekolo Mahlangu-Ngcobo is a native of South Africa. She is the first black South African to receive a Doctor of Ministry degree.

While in South Africa she taught at Seoding Elementary school. She also trained as a nurse and midwife at Baragwanath Hospital and attended University of North (Turfloop) to study a Diploma in Nursing Education. Her education was interrupted by her political activism around Steve Biko's death.

She has been involved in anti-Apartheid movements in South Africa and in exile (Canada and U.S.A.). She was detained and held in solitary confinement in South Africa.

She fled South Africa in 1980 and came to the United States of America in 1981. She was able to return to South Africa in 1991 to lead the National Coordinating Council for Repatriation (NCCR) of South African Exiles.

She was called to the ministry in 1988. She was ordained an itinerant elder in the African Methodist Episcopal church in 1992.

In 1997, Rev. Dr. Mahlangu-Ngcobo went to Liberia to lead a workshop on Conflict Management for Women and also to observe the National Election under the auspices of The Organization of African Unity.

In the U.S. she received four degrees: Bachelor of Science degree (Magna Cum Laude) from Morgan State University; Master of Public Health from The Johns Hopkins University; Master of Arts from St. Mary's University and Seminary; Doctor of Ministry (Samuel D. Proctor Fellow) from United Theological Seminary.

Rev. Dr. Mankekolo Mahlangu-Ngcobo was one of 35 members of the District of Columbia HIV Prevention Community Planning Committee, appointed by the Commissioner of Public Health in Washington, D.C. for 2 years (1994-1995). The committee was a collaboration between the government and the community created for the purpose of ensuring that the HIV prevention needs of the citizens of the District of

Columbia were represented and addressed.

She has written five books, namely, *The Preaching of Bishop John R. Bryant,* (1992), *100 Ways of Empowering Women,* (1996), *To God be the Glory: Celebration of the Life of Bishop Frederick Calhoun James,* (1996), *Wise Words – Men Empowering Men,* (1998), and *Women in the Ministry: Their Trials and Triumphs,* (2000). *AIDS in Africa: The African and Prophetic Perspective* (2001) is her 6th book.

She is a former A.M.E. Washington Conference Coordinator of Women in the Ministry.

She was on the ministerial staff of Metropolitan A.M.E. in Washington, D.C., where she led the Women's Ministry and Single Ministry at Metropolitan A.M.E. Church. She was also on the ministerial staff at Bethel A.M.E. Church in Baltimore, Maryland, prior to joining Metropolitan.

Rev. Dr. Mankekolo Mahlangu-Ngcobo is the former Co-Chair of the Maryland delegation to the Summit on Africa and presently is the President Emeritus of Association of Maryland African Society. (AMAS) She is also a board member of the Sub-Sahara Relief Fund Inc. (SSRF), and a member of the Religious Action Network of the African Action.

She is an adjunct professor at Morgan University and Sojourner Douglass College in Baltimore, Maryland, teaching Health and Religion and Health courses.

Rev. Dr. Mankekolo Mahlangu-Ngcobo is Founder and Pastor of a new church, Kalafong A.M.E. Mission Church in Baltimore, Maryland. Kalafong is a Southern African word, which means, "A Healing Place" for individuals, families, communities and nations through Christ who strengthens us.

ORDERING INFORMATION

Name _____

Church/Org./Bus _____

Street Address _____

City/State/Zip Code _____

Phone: (   ) _____

The Preaching of Bishop John R. Bryant ____ x $12.50 = $ _____

100 Ways of Empowering Women _____ x $10.00 = $ _____

*To God Be the Glory: Celebration of the Life
of Bishop Frederick Calhoun James* _____ x $15.95 = $ _____

Wise Words: Men Empowering Men _____ x $7.95 = $ _____

*Women in the Ministry:
Their Trials and Their Triumphs* _____ x $12.50 = $ _____

*AIDS in Africa: The African and
the Prophetic Perspective* _____ x $19.50 = $ _____

Maryland Residents add 5% sales tax)
Shipping and handling: $3.00 for first book,
$.75 for each additional   Total = $_____

Make check or money order payable to:
Rev. Dr. Mankekolo Mahlangu-Ngcobo. Allow 2-4 for delivery.

Mail Orders to:
Rev. Dr. Mankekolo Mahlangu-Ngcobo
PO Box 29776
Baltimore, MD 21216
email: Mankekolo@aol.com
Bookstore/Wholesale inquiries, please call or FAX (410) 233-4649